Yoga and Optimum Health After 40

Yoga and Optimum Health After 40

Yvonne Alexander Seltzer

Writer's Showcase

San Jose   New York   Lincoln   Shanghai

Yoga and Optimum Health After 40

Writer's Showcase
an imprint of iUniverse.com, Inc.

For information address:
iUniverse.com, Inc.
5220 S 16th, Ste. 200
Lincoln, NE 68512
www.iuniverse.com

Note: This book is not intended as a medical tome. See your personal care person for medical problems.

ISBN: 0-595-18912-1

Printed in the United States of America

A DOCTOR COMMENTS

"THE AUTHOR SPELLS OUT THE WAYS THAT YOGA IS GOOD FOR HEALTH. IN THIS ARTFULLY WRITTEN BOOK, SHE TELLS YOU HOW TO DO IT". WALTER BORTZ, M.D., PALO ALTO MEDICAL FOUNDATION, AUTHOR OF BOOKS "WE LIVE TOO SHORT AND DIE TOO LONG" AND "DARE TO BE 100".

YOGA RALLIES PATIENT WITH CRITICAL ILLNESS

A YOUNG DOCTOR SAID THE MAGIC WORD, 'YOGA' AFTER YEARS OF TREATMENT FOR SPINAL DISK DEPLETION, FIBROMYALGIA, CHRONIC MYOFASCIAL PAIN SYNDROME, AND DEPRESSION. I FINALLY LISTENED TO MY AUNT YVONNE SELTZER AND BEGAN LIFE AGAIN "IN HARMONY WITH YOGA".

LYNETTE GAGNON, OLYMPIA, WA., SCHOOL TEACHER

The cover picture is a symbol
of the breath of life.
Life is a circle. When earth
breathes, there is life.
You are earth, your breath
is life. Your breath is
the flower of life.

Amy Seltzer

CONTENTS

This book is dedicated to our son Kent.....

The light and the spirit endure.

Acknowledgements

This book would never have been published without the help of the following people: first, my husband and agent, Harry K. Seltzer, a man of great energies and enduring enthusiasms and one who never gives up. My special thanks to Pamela Alexander Auld, who nurtured the book from its beginnings and to Patrick, Mary and Birge Seltzer. Katherine Alexander Anderson, Tracy Alexander Brulotte, and Lynette Alexander Gagnon, always there with words I wanted to hear.

Thanks also to Peggy Morrow, Nutritionist, and Linda Zecca, my Yoga teacher, for editorial expertise in their respective fields and caring support always. My appreciation also to Duane Kaemmerling, Mary Ellen Heising, Luther Nichols, and Meredith Brokaw, special counsel at critical times.

Finally, merci beaucoup to the faithful friends and colleagues in the rooting section: Bob La Fontaine, Liane Bagnall, Father Larry Kambitsch, Joan and John Smits, Charles and Dixie Briggs, Lou Bryant, John Sullivan, Gene and Jane Klecan, Joe Morrow, Phil O'Brien, Sally Hitchman, Pat D'Alessandro, Brian Murtha, Esq., James Engleman, M.D., Walter Bortz, M.D., Stephen Plager, M.D. F.A.C.S., Carson Kelly, C. Jean Poulos, Ph.D. our excellent word processors, Christy Marani, Amy Neiblum and Candice Gabrio. Lastly, Owen Norman for his important early assistance.

FOREWORD

The mission of "Yoga and Optimum Health After 40" is to focus greater public awareness on a more positive view of aging through exercise—in this case, yoga, a powerful, proven answer to aging.

This is not only a book about yoga for older people. It is a book that promotes the idea of healthy aging, by a lay person who has read widely and deeply on the subject for years; one who has observed herself and many others in the aging process and has thought long thoughts about it. One who has said, "Yes" to dealing with the process, all the while questioning, questing...

Aging is a challenge just as adolescence is a challenge or the child-bearing/child rearing years and working years are challenges. The significant difference with aging is in its built-in, mostly unacknowledged handicap in the public mind: the people involved in the process are, in a word, OLD.

In the American mind, this is almost the unforgivable sin: Old is ugly, decrepit, helpless, crabby, infirm and boring to much of the public and a good slice of the medical profession. And when it happens to you (and it will, it will; if you're lucky) and you suffer that first humiliating discrimination, you wonder why. Naturally do you wonder: here you are, the person you have always been—except you're older (or you look older) and for probably the first time in your life some one is treating you like a second class citizen or worse.

No person escapes. I have witnessed so accomplished a person as Walter Cronkite humiliated in front of an audience of millions by a usually decent anchorman asking what he has been doing with his time since CBS forced his retirement. Cronkite, gracious and sharp as ever, obviously slightly taken aback, set the man straight. Seventy-five plus, still working—writing, producing and originating creative, educational television shows on the Discovery Channel, still sailing his beloved boat, Walter Cronkite is living a full, productive life that eminently suits him, as are many elders.

So the aging American faces this difficult challenge with a handicap somewhat reminiscent of the public attitude toward returned Vietnam veterans: vast public disinterest in the problem, contempt for the person's current place in society and discrimination based on a perceived powerlessness to change.

The answer to such a dilemma is to fight: For health, for self-respect and the respect of the broader society. Reality tells the aging person to summon up those American pioneering instincts (not the blood-thirsty ones—the survival ones) and fight this last battle. Unfortunately, many of us do not like reality, no matter what our age.

Simply observing older people demonstrates that there are as many ways to age as there are people. Some of us are aware of no handicaps of any kind. We all know others who are 'old' at 35 and remain that way until the end. The spectrum runs the gamut: denial; complete surrender; with all manner of reactions between those poles.

The fight to maintain wellness, self-respect and enhanced quality of life among elders has a powerful and ancient ally in yoga. Yoga is a giant step toward engagement with life for any person. Its effects are deceptively quiet and potent for anyone. For elders it can work profound change.

1. Yoga raises energy: do all you want to do in your life, whether it is a cause you believe in, a desire to help children or other people, or an absorbing hobby. Yoga gives you the energy to engage life.

2. The increased well-being brought about by yoga makes life pleasurable, no matter what the age. Well-being is a priceless asset you can give yourself through yoga. It adds grace and joy to your days.

3. Yoga preserves your looks and your body shape. It has noticeable cosmetic effects that cost nothing more than your motivation to persist, and improves rather than harms the whole body. Plastic surgery is invasive but quick. Yoga is not.

The integrity of the facial muscle structure is striking in long-time yoga practitioners. Facial features do not change as much in the aging process: the face will not sag, eyes remain natural and sparkling, skin tone is enhanced by improved circulation. A look and air of youthfulness and zest is common in such people.

Posture improves, and as it does, years roll off your appearance. Muscles throughout the upper trunk, back, legs and balance muscles strengthen, promoting an easy, graceful posture.

All of these factors combine to build confidence and lightness toward life and people.

Yoga is what works!

Introduction

Yoga and Optimum Health is designed for the older beginner in yoga and as a supplement for those already enrolled in such a class. It is also suited for people of all ages who are newcomers to adaptive yoga practice.

No person is too old for yoga; those people whose physical condition might restrict demanding postures may safely do the relaxation, breathing practices and energy-increasing techniques.

The yoga student, through gentle but persistent practice of postures, relaxation and breathing, is introduced to a new level of physical and mental awareness, of stretching the self to subtle limits previously unknown.

This inner self, physical and mental, is awakened in many people for the first time, after age 55. In fact, in India, where it originated, yoga is not started in many cases until age 50; in that Eastern country, it is believed that at a younger age, the person is too immature to benefit fully.

In a yoga class, the body, particularly the lungs, heart, muscles and nervous system is truly freed to escape the wear and tear, the pressures of today's society; and the participant comes to enjoy a period of peace and relaxation that are tremendous life-enhancers.

Yoga stimulates faith in one's innate constructive healing powers, as feelings of bodily well-being take hold with continued practice. These feelings of well-being in turn work in a cumulative way to increase a positive attitude, one of the basic tenets of yoga. I have seen the miracle happen time after time: when muscles are toned and the whole-body circulation is improved, sluggish attitudes make a shift steadily toward positiveness and trust in the life process. This attitude shift alone is a tremendous boon to people over 40, especially when they are just beginning to deal with an unfriendly social climate.

In learning yoga through this book and in yoga class, our goal is wellness and peace. And the enjoyment of life's many blessings.

Yvonne Alexander Seltzer

Special Note:

Shortly before deadline, "Beginning Again in Harmony With Yoga" arrived.

A true story by my niece, Lynette Gagnon of Olympia, Washington, it appears on the following page.

I believe you will find it intriguing, shocking perhaps and provocative. If only for Lynette's use of the beautiful word *harmony* in conjunction with Yoga, I would have thought to include it. But there is so much more......

Beginning Again in Harmony with Yoga

I was celebrating my twenty-first birthday when my wondrous Aunt Yvonne first introduced me to yoga. She sent me a picture of herself standing on her head in her leotard to illustrate the balance and energy that the practice exemplified. She was about 50 then and in her second bloom. Of course, being twenty-something and a zealous overachiever, I didn't think I needed anything for balance or energy. Besides, I thought she was a little crazy to be standing on her head at 50!

Years passed. As my godmother, Yvonne never forgot my birthday or succinct remark on the benefits of yoga. Sometimes she'd visit and put my sister and me through breathing and stretching exercises. Like a slow, gentle drip the message began to saturate my consciousness. Yoga was good stuff! But I still didn't feel the need!

More years passed. I gave birth to my two children using LaMaze, adopted a Down's Syndrome child, founded and directed a mid-size day-care center, and taught for another 20 years. Still, I had no idea how to make time for myself. But dear Yvonne continued the gentle nudging routine. About the time my children left for college, I was in an automobile accident in which I suffered a severe whiplash injury. After chiropractory, physical therapy, massage therapy, and extensive pain medication, I still could hardly move. I was diagnosed with Spinal Disk Depletion, Fibromyalgia, Chronic Myofascial Pain Syndrome, and Depression. My weight was up to 190, which was way more than my five-foot frame should carry.

Thank God I had a young doctor who was skilled in complementary medicine. He said the magic word, "YOGA"! Now I indeed had the need, and all those years of sweet suggestions by Yvonne Seltzer came tumbling back into my consciousness. It took me six months or so of trying different approaches, teachers, and schedules. Finally, I found a class that matched my needs at the Olympia Community Yoga Center with Ray A Grace. Mr. Grace uses his years of yoga study and a thorough knowledge of human anatomy, along with a talent for vivid imagery, to guide us in our practice of yoga.

After two years of yoga class twice a week, I'm still just beginning to listen to my body. From the little that I've learned so far, I have gained vast benefits. I have been able to reduce my pain medications drastically. Regular yoga has enabled me to separate and manipulate my own vertebrae, lengthen my tendons and ligaments, so that bones and muscles aren't pinching nerves. Yoga is my ever-present chiropractor. Frequent use of the asanas has strengthened and tightened my muscles and tissues. I have gone from a size eighteen to a size eight over a two-year period with little loose skin or body shock. My weight has dropped from 190 to 135 pounds. Frequent yoga serves as my physical and massage therapist. When I leave a yoga class, I feel like I can fly! Nothing seems impossible!

Around 50, if you are lucky, you have reached the time of life when you know how to listen, really listen, to all those quiet voices inside. Your body is longing for a change from the breathtaking pace to a breathing space. Your soul yearns for wise silence.

Now, you are ready to make time for yourself. If you are reading this, you are also fortunate to have an angel whispering in your ear, named Yvonne Seltzer. Listen and begin again-in harmony with yoga!

Lynette Gagnon-

Genesis 6:3 says,

"…And the Lord said…man's days shall be a hundred and twenty years."

CHAPTER 1

What is Yoga?

The word yoga derives from a 5,000 year old Sanskrit word meaning "union" or "to yoke together". It is an apt description of the practice of yoga on a daily basis, where the aim is to unite the body, mind, and spirit through the physical exercises or asanas, combined with meditation and positive thinking.

Yoga is a natural system based on the connection between breath, mind and body; a natural system and practice that promotes optimum health. It is truly impossible to practice yoga under a good teacher for a few weeks, months or years and not have your body, mind, spirit, and nerves feel lighter, healed, uplifted. Yoga is not a religion, and it is not occult, or beyond the normal in any way.

As Yogi William Zorn has said, it is an antidote to the unnatural and high pressure life that most people live today. Zorn learned his yoga as a war prisoner. It saved his sanity.

It is a fact: yoga works! Through regular practice, with increased awareness, you will begin to know and deeply respect the person inside you: to learn to love life, to say Yes! to life.

CHAPTER 2

The Benefits of Yoga

STRETCHING THE SELF

Americans are living longer now than at any previous time in history. At the same time, burnout is a big problem in this country at all adult age levels. Younger adults often burn out from too much activity and not enough emphasis on sleep, exercise and enjoyment of life. Conversely, older people experience burnout from apathy and inactivity, a faint-hearted unwillingness to test their mettle, physically and mentally. Such attitudes in older people are seductive and widespread in our society. Their seductiveness is implicit in being human, and buying into current attitudes toward aging. Needless fear, apprehension and depression are for these reasons pervasive in large segments of the older population in this country.

Yoga is especially suitable for people over 40, because it immediately promotes a positive sense of well being. The breathing exercises are an important part of this renewed vital sense, as are the benefits of total relaxation and the gentle stretching and toning of long-idle muscles.

Aches and pains dampen enjoyment of life; to fight back not once, but as often as needed, is to defeat our society's wrong-headed concept of age as helplessness. To this purpose yoga works systematically on every part of the body and raises the general standard of health. The student becomes a more whole person; a more competent person; in short and in fact, a more joyful person.

In the words of Sr. Mary Martin Weaver, a Catholic nun featured in Parade Magazine, "People have gotten flabby, and I don't mean just physically. Anything that's too much, people just don't want to do. Thing is, there are no rewards unless you try. Age should never be a barrier to full participation in life. A good diet's important. Exercise is important. But what's most important is to enjoy life to its fullest, to do things for others and never, ever be afraid to stretch your limits." Sr. Weaver is not a yoga student but is a prize winner in the Senior Olympics who had never done any athletics until age 55. She has been a prize winning ice skater for 10 years. [Parade Magazine, July 15, 1990].

We must dismiss the thought 'too old!' so widespread in society that every one of us over 40 is tempted to believe it at times of fatigue and discouragement.

WE MUST GO FOR IT!

YOGA, AGING AND WELLNESS

Yoga is a way to dramatically change ideas of what women and men over 40 can do, can be and can accomplish. It demolishes ill-founded, stubborn prejudices about aging that prevent people over 40 from living full, satisfying lives. No matter what your age or physical condition, yoga can help you in some way to feel better, stronger and more relaxed and at peace with yourself and your world. Yoga works!

It has been well said that one must rebuild one's confidence regularly throughout life. Confidence is crucial at mid-life and beyond. Yoga builds confidence while aiming for wellness. Wellness is defined as peak mental and physical condition.

Yoga builds wellness and confidence with a three-pronged effect: increased physical strength plus deep mental and physical relaxation. In addition, yoga breathing increases stamina, balances and integrates the muscle systems, the nervous system and the circulation throughout in people over 40. A sense of well-being is key to confidence, ease, and enjoyment of life. Yoga builds both through breathing; the asanas; and a positive attitude.

Yoga asanas (postures) are the quintessential preventative medicine: increased circulation and increased flexibility plus a sense of well-being means better mobility, better memory, plus awakened curiosity and interest in life.

In fact, to repeat, self-care through yoga almost immediately heightens the sense of physical well-being in people of any age. A deep sense of satisfaction stems from the power inherent in self-help. The power of self-help lights an internal fire often extinguished by lack of awareness; or in many cases an uncaring, if not punitive, attitude toward one's own body, both common attitudes in this country, with its history of Puritanism which is here in subtle ways even in 2000. In addition, American men in many instances labor under a macho ethic that ignoring physical discomfort is a positive good, a sign of manliness; self-defeating though such ideas may be, they are difficult for men to confront or soften.

In the case of women, recent studies show that they are under-diagnosed for early cancer by male physicians and that male physicians no matter what their age, leave 40% of their older women patients unaware that yearly mammograms are mandatory for women after age 40. In addition, women of all ages are under-diagnosed and under-treated for heart attacks by physicians. Not only at the beginning of heart disease, but throughout its course in women patients, it is under-treated.

These attitudes and facts should alert us to take a realistic, responsible interest in the body, and to make good, responsible self-care a serious pursuit in the second half of life.

BREATHING FOR POWER AND RELAXATION

Most people over 40 have inhibited and ineffective breathing patterns due to the accumulated trauma and stress of daily life. These breathing problems are deeply involuntary and unconscious in nature. Stressed breathing affects the brain and thus the whole body. Many people are consequently under-oxygenated; (i.e. the blood does not receive enough oxygen to enable the body to function efficiently). Proper breathing techniques can bring a powerful charge of energy into the body to heal, strengthen resistance to disease and stress, help rid the body and bloodstream of toxins and thereby activate the body's wonderful regenerative processes. Toxins are another name for free radicals, a by-product of oxidation. Oxidation is a process much like rusting, that turns fats in the bloodstream into alien deposits that build up in the walls of blood vessels and arteries. The scientific community is at work in many places studying the role of free radicals in health and disease.

Yoga breathing techniques work also at the psychological level, putting us in touch with our real selves and our real agenda, in time. The brain becomes what it does, and with yoga breathing techniques, the breath 'clears' the brain, and usually in short order. This clarity results in a distinct feeling of lightness throughout the body and brain. Increased awareness of self and others and of the total life environment happens in those people who are open to it.

In addition, proper breathing while bringing extra stores of oxygen to the blood, also stimulates the brain, releasing creative energies. People over 40 need this. It is an "oxygen high," in other words: effective, harmless, and life enhancing.

Does your spirit feel old as the sea; aggrieved, beat-down? Yoga will help you heal it. For those over 40 who are interested in spiritual development, proper breathing also works at the spiritual level, helping such men and women to discover their true purpose here on our planet. Yoga has worked in this way for thousands of years. It is a proven system of physical, psychological and spiritual wellness.

With yoga, change your mind, change your life is a reality; a comfortable, energized, joyful second half of life is yours.

Yoga adds to quality of life after 40 in many ways.

According to the National Institutes of Health Study on Aging the quality of life in older people includes the following; the ability to think, feel, interact with others, work, enjoy recreational activities, engage in sexual behaviors, be able to move about, practice one's religious beliefs, have a degree of independence in daily living and make choices for oneself about the course of one's life:

Major purpose of this report from the National Institutes of Health (first by this respected scientific body) is to dissuade health professionals from the belief that growing old necessarily means growing frail. Health care professionals should collaborate with exercise specialists, according to the report, to develop programs in exercise counseling, promotion and instruction, in other words, a team approach to health in older people, rather than the fragmented one that now prevails. Perhaps it is time for people over 40 to consider a team approach to health. It is an approach that makes sense.

"Self-health care is the future," says Faith Popcorn, researcher, "...in the end we've all got to take care of ourselves. We're each inside our body alone and the final responsibility is our own".

A key to prevention of most diseases is practicing a healthy lifestyle with attention to diet and cholesterol levels, exercise, stress reduction and avoiding smoking and excessive drinking. Fitness measures work for young and old, according to nurse/newspaper columnist Virginia Shiras,

R.N. and Isadore Rosenfeld, M.D., author of **Modern Prevention, the New Medicine.**

Diagnosis and treatment are the doctor's main concern, say both Shiras and Rosenfeld, but each person must take responsibility for learning what he or she must do to stay well, active, alert and mentally engaged with life. As Shiras says, "by following healthful lifestyles and being aware of one's health, many serious health problems can be avoided".

Prevention does work. And often it is a matter of common sense and simple procedures.

Inactivity at any age is bad; in older people it is a killer. It can cause muscle tension, emotional instability, poor appetite and bowel problems, to begin a short list. Muscles are meant to be used. Unused, they accumulate tension from bodily reactions to fear, anxiety, anger and frustration. Unless discharged through the means of exercise, this tension builds, directly affecting emotional well-being.

A healthy lifestyle plus yoga makes a dynamic combination for optimum health in the second half of life.

The feeling of inner power engendered by self-help (or I prefer the term self-motivation) is crucial to the good life for people over 40. According to the report of the National Institutes of Health previously quoted, "Prolonged well-being is the goal for those over 50." Yoga fills this goal abundantly.

There is little evidence that the health of older persons is of interest to the general public, or even to the medical establishment, another factor that should push us to a grass-roots approach to health care. I do not make such a statement lightly. Having observed first-hand the shocking slipshod care at times given older people in my own family, and having spoken to numbers of elders on this subject, I can verify it from personal experience. Ability to pay seems to have no bearing on the quality of care; health care is not medical care: health care involves social and political issues.

The mere fact that there are few books in circulation written on the subject of how to stay well while aging, is telling. A recent survey of a couple of thriving book stores in Santa Cruz County, CA brought a look of puzzlement on the clerk's face when asked, "Where is your shelf of books on aging located in the store?" *Two* books were in stock on the subject, in each store. What former Governor Richard Lamm of Colorado has called "the most significant demographic event of our lifetime; the aging of America and the aging of the aged," has been largely ignored in medicine and in society as a whole. My feeling is that the situation will not be remedied in any significant fashion until the Baby Boom generation is in its late fifties. They make more noise than most generations, and hopefully Boomers will be prolific writers and activists on aging. At this juncture, becoming informed, taking personal responsibility and having a grass roots activism about personal health is the only way to counteract the oversights in U.S. health care for older people.

A healthy lifestyle, plus yoga makes a dynamic combination for health in the second half of life. True, it does take motivation—more motivation than perhaps most people think they can muster—to begin yoga practice and to stay with a program until one has mastered a number of asanas and can practice alone.

An additional value of yoga classes for over 40 cohorts is the prevention of social isolation. In a yoga class, energy is transmitted to all participants in the class from the teacher to class members, members to teacher and to each other. A yoga class is perceptibly more charged and relaxed at its end than when it first gathers.

Walter Bortz, M.D. currently with the Palo Alto Medical Foundation, Palo Alto, California has said that "Exercise is the balance wheel to tension," in his book, *We Live Too Short and We Die Too Long*. Bortz, a runner, decries the inactivity of most people over 40. He has studied primitive African tribes whose members run at least 35 miles per day to obtain food. He found superb arterial systems in the Africans he studied and began running himself.

In the case of the writer, I turned to yoga after a horrendous trauma at age 34 that had left me a changed person physically, mentally and spiritu-

ally. Before, I had been confident, strong and well, a lover of life and people. I was now, seven years later, fearful, ailing a lot and wanting desperately again to be as I once was. Physically and mentally I had changed in
ways I did not like. Spiritually I had changed in ways I did like and
wanted to solidify and integrate into a wholeness that had eluded me.

One of the prime targets I was aiming for was help with the tension
that now seemed to be part of a busy life. I enrolled in a yoga class at the
local Civic Center, and found to my amazement that the teacher, Charles
Horn, was a man in his 70's...with the vigor, enthusiasm and flexibility of
a much younger person.

I soon found that yoga does much more than help diffuse muscular
tension, as most exercise does. In Hatha yoga, which is the physical postures system of yoga, the body's muscles, bones, joints, organs, glands,
nerves and myriad cells are deliberately manipulated, stretched and
relaxed in a daily process.

Yoga affects not only the physical body; the etheric body is engaged.
Deepak Chopra, M.D., a medical doctor and Ayurveda practitioner has
said that the bio-chemistry of the body is the by-product of our awareness.
This conclusion makes eminent sense to a person who has practiced yoga
consistently over a few years. It is self-evident to such a person. The etheric
body, so called by the alternative healing profession, comprises the subtle
energy of the body, the energy field that interpenetrates the dense physical
body. It is this body field, quite malleable, that holds keys to healing and
to well being. It is a body field that each one of us knows is as real as the
universe and as mysterious. We can activate, influence, cherish and
enhance this mysterious body. Yoga is the key.

Dr. Allen Barbour, former chief of the Stanford University Diagnostic
Clinic and much honored as a clinical teacher, that is one who is in the
trenches with his patients, has for 40 years been exploring the influence of
life stress on wellness. His research found over this long time that only
one-third of his patients could be diagnosed as having organic disease.
Another one-third had symptoms but no organic cause, which symptoms

he felt resulted from stress and ongoing problems in the patient's life. The final third group of Dr. Barbour's patients, followed in over 40 years of research, were ill with a combination of organic and stress-related disease. His conclusions after a lifetime of study are worth consideration by any thoughtful person over 40 who wants to stay well. Particularly interesting is his finding that while psychosomatic illness and pain are real, such pain is not easily treatable by current medical methods. He is the author of a book, *Caring for Patients, A Critique of the Medical Model*, published in 1994 by Stanford University Press.

Stress and tension are perhaps more than anything else, the "bad dragon" of Western life style. Many people over 40 have struggled with this dragon for decades. It affects their personalities, their mood, permeates their life. To these people tension is often more than anything else a fight to gain control over an enemy that threatens peace of mind, suffuses every facet of life, and in the end, affects their health.

Yoga offers a peaceful way to deal with tension: assimilate it into your life instead of fighting it, for it is the conflict inherent in fighting the tension that causes it to continue, in cyclical fashion. Disarm and assimilate tension by simply doing yoga exercises and learning the breathing and relaxation; gradually, the bad dragon of tension is tamed: with perseverance on the student's part, it shrivels in size, then disappears. After the first three yoga classes, the student will notice an immediate improvement in tension level—it may be slight, but it will be real. The reality is that you do not even have to have a goal to reduce tension—just remain open to the postures, do them; do the relaxation; try the breathing even if you are awkward at it: a more relaxed body and mind are assured.

According to yoga, body, mind and spirit are one. The yogi believes that the mind is present throughout the cells of the body and is not just in the brain field. So that when the yoga adept stretches the muscles, strengthens, energizes and relaxes the body, and does yoga breathing or meditation, the mind is affected in subtle but profound ways.

The breath controls the life force: where the life force is diminished, aging begins. Deep breathing techniques bring stores of oxygen to the bloodstream, and every vital organ, endocrine gland, nerve center and body tissue is bathed in nourishment. Correct breathing means staying young longer.

Deep breathing combined with the asanas also affects the glands. The endocrine glands, the pituitary and pineal glands in the head (the pineal gland is the "master gland" of the body.) Thyroid and para-thyroid in the throat; the adrenal glands set above the kidneys; the sex glands, ovaries in women, testes in men, all have vital work to do that is positively affected by yoga practice.

Meditation, a simple breathing technique that seems mysterious because of its name and is in truth mysterious in its effects to most people, has been studied by Dr. Herbert Benson of Harvard, who has written a book The Relaxation Response. Meditation can offer an additional healing tool for the mind and spirit akin to that which exercise (the asanas) does for the body.

These are subtle concepts and only in the experience of them will some people believe their power. Yoga and meditation are more experiential than intellectual. While such subtle ideas may seem sound even to the uninitiated, it is in doing them that the simplicity, yet the historically proven soundness, is grasped by the student.

The rhythms of yoga echo the rhythms of life—the rhythm of the universe, of the sea, of the animal world. Both the circadian and ultradian rhythms of women's and men's lives reverberate in yoga and meditation.

Part 1

HEALTH PROBLEMS OF AGING

CHAPTER 3

Stress

A recent spiritual memoir by a well known Northern California author recounts in detail long months spent in a program where she learned to eat when hungry instead of stuffing food into her mouth at rote meal times or when stress pushed her eating habits over the edge. Charles Horn, my first yoga teacher, would call this a horror story.

Hunger pangs get lost and confused in the emotional jungles of men and women pressured by constant hurry, sleep deprivation, long work hours without any kind of sensible break and nightmare commutes. Hunger is vital, natural but in a badly stressed person hunger sometimes becomes the enemy; and obsessive need to be filled replaces it.

Stress is thus a major cause of over-eating and poor nutrition and this is only one of the bad effects.

Research released in the past 3 months has established that women feel stress more than men, at all ages and under similar life circumstances. Not surprisingly, working women with children are the most stressed of all humans on the planet. This is not a U.S. phenomenon; the careful research was conducted world wide with a sample of 30,000 people.

While most men are able to shed stress when they leave the workplace, women's stress levels stay elevated long after they leave the office or plant.

In addition to stress at work and home women's stress has Catch 22 aspects, sometimes self-imposed: i.e. women push themselves to live up to expectations–sometimes their own (a tough one!). Sometimes other people's (can be equally tough). Relationships, family and social cause stress in women. Men are not nearly as vulnerable to relationship stress. Physical appearance is a stressor to women, not to men. Tied in with appearance, food and weight problems stress women, as well. It is a rare male who worries about appearance or overweight.

People over 40 who experience grief, loss or trauma, those who retire early or late and those who must deal with chronic illness are many times in great pain. Almost all kinds of pain causes stress; pain effects vary from person to person. Keep in mind also that for every five years one adds to a person's life it takes a longer time to recuperate from physical stress such as accidents, surgery and injury. Yoga helps such people by keeping alive the spark of hope in the spirit and mind. Keeping the body physical systems operating well is a great help in functioning better and working through grief and other severe mental pain. A physically energized system helps to alleviate fear in fearful persons and aids anxious or irritable ones to function more peacefully.

Journal writing is tremendously helpful also. It can be a very powerful experience to record your darkest thoughts as they occur. Put all the pain, confusion and fear on paper as best you can. This exercise can be very releasing. The act of writing integrates the mind-body connection. Journal writing also releases a creative impulse that most people experience as a healing force infusing the body and calming the mind. A journal writing friend who is a yoga teacher reports that she often experiences a real change in perspective for the better when she has finished writing. The act of writing calms fears. Once set down, fear can often be faced with courage. Rather than let the fears of distress stew along in the mind, the process of releasing fear can begin, with you.

If you are badly stressed I would advise you seriously consider journaling. You learn what you do and writing one's experiences has a more profound effect than most people can imagine. If you can hold a pencil, you can write no matter what your age–6 to 106; write your pain away. In a lot of people, stress is a synonym for misery and journaling helps relieve misery in the very act of writing.

Try it!

If the above stress busters do not appeal to you (after all, we are all different) there are other means of relief available.

Music is wonderful-flood the house or room with it. So is massage. Deep breathing and meditation have already been mentioned. Support groups can help and so can planned family discussion times.

More formal stress relief is yours if you invest time with an able psychologist, psychiatrist; some priests and ministers are trained counselors. I have friends and relatives who although of neither belief have been well counseled by Rabbi's, and by Buddhist teachers. Whatever the issue, a professional perspective can be very helpful in resolving stress and discovering the path to peace.

CHAPTER 4

Depression

One of the very real threats to well-being in older people is depression. In depression, the mind, body and spirit are affected..."the disabling effects were comparable to those of a serious heart condition...Only arthritis was judged to be more painful, and only serious heart conditions resulted in more days in bed," according to the National Institute of Health Study on Aging.

My feeling is that most people regard depression as scary and mysterious. People who have depression are not weird. They are *sick* and when they have a severe depression they are VERY SICK. In reality, it is a disease, as high blood pressure is, or heart disease or cancer. As they are, it is caused by physiological, metabolic, genetic and psychological forces within the individual. As they do, its victims do better with recovery when diagnosed early. Unlike them, this disease has been stigmatized by superstition, and because of this, older people especially tend to delay getting help. I would alert you, that if you are feeling 'down' or blue (seriously so) for over two weeks, accompanied by weight loss, sleep problems, or unusual irritability and inability to concentrate, seek help. In most people, depression is not chronic.

Depression certainly stems from a homeostatic imbalance. Homeostasis is the balance or equilibrium of the inner body and is dependent in part upon the proper levels of catecholamines (adrenaline and noradrenaline) in certain areas of the brain. Anti- depressant drugs help by evening out the brain chemical levels. Balanced levels of catecholamines in the brain and throughout the body organize the human body's response to work.

Interestingly enough, psychiatrists have found that exercise (which is work for the body) is a very effective treatment for depression. In that regard, the physiological response to reactivating a lethargic human body is instructive: the heart rate increases, the lungs stretch, blood vessels are dilated, fuels for energy turn at-the-ready; all systems Go! Those marvelous catecholamines are at work once more.

Conversely, Russian space scientists have observed that healthy young cosmonauts, forced into inactivity by their mission, become depressed. It becomes clear, after not too much logical thought, that depression is yet another illness linked to inactivity.

In fact, Dr. Walter Bortz has set forth the idea that since man for eons and eons has needed constant physical activity to stay well, the inactivity of this society of couch potatoes may mean that our entire society is depressed. Think about it! A depressing idea. But given the violence and drug abuse in our society (irrational acts on their face) not completely off the wall.

Samuel Butler said, "The more a thing knows its own mind, the more living (alive) it becomes". In other words, in many ways, awareness and a deep sense of who you are as a person is the key to making life healthier and thus easier to live and to enjoy. Exercise physiologists tell us that awareness of a muscle will allow you to use it and that stretching a muscle brings it into awareness. So it is with the self within. If a person over 40 does not know how wellness feels (i.e. if he is not aware that there are options to feeling ill or depressed) he/she may spend what has been called The Third Age, (that time after youth and middle age) in a vegetative state. An educational program stressing the need for physical and mental activity is badly needed in this country, aimed at the over-40 demographic.

The brain becomes what it does. In the recovery phase of depression (and in prevention also) yoga postures can help get the catecholamines working, with the asanas and the breathing. Yoga breathing may help awaken the powers of concentration which struggle mightily in depression. And the discipline of a fixed stance for each posture surely helps concentration. When physical practice is combined with medication and therapy, the prognosis is excellent.

Self-help plus support from professionals works.

The National Institute of Mental Health (NIMH) is a government agency that offers free information on depression and other mental disorders. For a NIMH publications list, write: NIMH Information Resources and Inquiries Branch, 5600 Fishers Lane, Rm. 7-02, Rockville, MD 20857. Or call the toll-free Depression Awareness Recognition, and Treatment (D/ART) number (1800-421-4211) for voicemail ordering information.

CHAPTER 5

Osteoporosis

A recent full page advertisement in a mass media news magazine shows a great looking, youthful woman with silvered hair. She is erect, graceful holding a robe just below her shoulders; pensive. "See how beautiful 60 can look?" the ad says. And below that: "See how invisible osteoporosis can be?"

This says it all. The woman may look vital, healthy. In fact, she is a deadly risk for osteoporosis.

Also called "brittle bone disease," osteoporosis in the recent past was the fourth leading killer of women; and yet very few women knew anything about it. That slowly may be changing. Detection, prevention and treatment of osteoporosis is part of a much welcomed, quiet revolution in women's health-care over the past 10 years. Technical and medical advances are part of the push, and people at risk for osteoporosis can now be tested for bone density. The test is a simple, pain-free, 15-minute, low-density X-ray procedure. At risk women and men can now be treated. The National Osteoporosis Foundation has stated that males are 20% of the 28 million people nationwide who have been diagnosed with the disease. Men make up one-third of those who break a hip, the most disabling of fractures. Wrists, legs, vertebrae and broken jaws are part of the scary list of the most common fractures in both men and women. Over-50 men are more at risk for such fractures than they are for developing prostate cancer, a fact which probably would surprise most people.

Before this women's health-care revolution, in the 'olden days' (five years ago in cyber-time) it safely could be predicted that one out of two women over 40 would suffer an osteoporotic fracture during her lifetime. Even today, this fact remains true for women over 50. The developmental pace of women's health-care has evolved so rapidly in these areas of medical research, prevention and treatment that the threat will vanish for informed women.

Even the US Congress has cooperated. The Federal government now subsidizes bone density screening for at risk women via Medicare, saving taxpayers millions in care and rehabilitation dollars. Breaking a bone at age 30 is an inconvenience, not a calamity. At most two months to recover. At seventy-plus a broken bone is serious, even full of dread. If the broken bone is a hip, prolonged bedrest follows. Such forced inactivity further weakens the injured person. Furthermore, a broken hip often requires rehabilitation so challenging for a 70-something person that patients often give up trying, slide into helplessness and die. This happened in my family. It was very, very expensive and too sad. The process took five agonizing years from the broken hip to death bed.

Once again, self-care strongly enters the picture. Studies indicate that bones better maintain their size and strength and density as we age, with regular exercise; that diet matters; that guided relaxation may matter.

How does osteoporosis start and how can we help ourselves to put it on the short list of disabling disease that is now defunct? Osteoporosis begins with a weakening of the skeletal bone mass, the superstructure of the body. The disease process weakens the skeletal foundation and eventually a bone breaks. Mild cases manifest with marked but limited posture change; in the more severely afflicted (80% of victims are elderly and female) the disease can lead to diminished height, caused by numerous small fractures along the spine. It contributes greatly to risk of falls and hip fractures in older women, and yoga can reduce that risk significantly, as it routinely protects against diseases of inflexibility and weak musculature.

Strong muscles throughout the body, a prime benefit of yoga practice, can better protect bones and joints in a fall, in addition to improving flexibility, mobility and balance. In addition, staying limber helps people keep up a wider range of activity which in itself is life-enhancing.

My first yoga teacher, Charles Horn, said those many years ago that all humans need fresh air, water and sun on their bodies every day. I believed him then and I believe him even more now: Sun, water and air on the body are wondrous life- enhancing gifts from the Creator of our universe to us and to all people since the dawn of time. Sun is vital also in helping to prevent osteoporosis, as the sun's ultraviolet rays act as catalyst in the body's absorption of Vitamin D. As with all else in this life, moderation is key with sunning.

Balance.

Think about it ...

With many delicious fruit yogurts, frozen and unfrozen, available now almost everywhere, there is very little excuse for not building calcium into the diet. Some fresh orange juices are calcium-fortified as well. Read the labels.

Common sense helps in keeping well. And yet many of us shun it. It's too cheap or not fast enough or easy enough for our many American couch potatoes.

At times in the past three years, I have been in a yoga class to which a woman in her early 70's was sent, part of her physiotherapist's prescription for battling a mild case of osteoporosis. I was delighted to talk to Jane enthusiastically about yoga and disappointed but not particularly surprised when she dropped out after three classes (excellently taught classes for people over 40, taught by Linda Zecca of Santa Cruz, CA) Linda, a caring teacher interested in wellness for older people, has been my teacher for the past eleven years.

I can't help but wonder how Jane is doing with her osteoporosis. Perhaps she is lifting weights, jumping rope or being faithful with meditation, deep breathing and relaxation, all of which help to cope with osteoporosis. I hope so. I know she was walking, which is excellent, but in itself not as good as a combination of muscle-strengthening practice along with walking.

Although calcium lack is specific for osteoporosis, most women do not realize that two factors are essential to metabolize calcium in women—estrogen and vitamin D. No matter how much calcium one consumes, it cannot be used by the body without these two critical elements.

In addition to building bones and skeleton, calcium is essential for the functioning of many body systems. It regulates blood pressure, heart rate and muscle contractions and when calcium dips below prime levels, the body takes the needed mineral from our bones, leading eventually into osteoporotic bones. Jay T. Kearney, a sports physiologist with the U.S. Olympic Committee in Colorado Springs, Colorado has said...."a muscle in use doesn't know if it's a Nautilus machine or push-ups or yoga that requires...strength..."(to perform a certain movement). The vital ingredient missing in Nautilus machines, push-ups and walking programs is hope. Yoga gives continually renewed hope, a potent natural medicine, to osteoporosis patients and other embattled humans. I have experienced this haunting, revelatory renewal of hope continually over my nearly 35 years of yoga practice. It kept me well after the loss of a much-loved son to drowning in a flash flood at age 22, when I was 52. I can honestly say that I do not think I would be alive today, much less well and energized, and positive, without yoga.

Dr. Walter Bortz, currently with the Palo Alto Medical Foundation, formerly of the Palo Alto Medical Clinic, has written that "the renewal capacity of life is one of its wonders." I would second that idea, adding that to be renewed you need hope. The process will not begin without hope. For women who already have developed "brittle bone disease", more options to limit the disease are available in 2000 than even two or three years ago. Yoga, along with other exercises; attention to nutrition with possible calcium diet supplements; and medication, all are helpful. Recent medical reports from university research facilities tell us that about 99% of calcium intake goes directly into the bones and teeth. A French study of the effects of calcium supplements combined with Vitamin A was reported late in 1993. That study involving 3,000 women of average age 84 (!) years found that supplement-provided women had 43% fewer hip fractures and 32% other fractures, specifically non-vertebral fractures, than women on placebos. An American doctor interested in osteoporosis, Richard Heaney, M.D. of Creighton University Medical School, also a calcium researcher, "estimates that the percent of such fractures prevented in the French study translates into 40,000 hip fractures in the United States per year." Fractures prevented could save one to two billion dollars a year in medical care. The suffering involved is almost unspeakable to a lay person, since these victims are in large part our most elderly, the 'old old'.

Unfortunately, most medical schools teach very little about nutrition and nothing about exercise, which Ruth Jacebowitz calls "the elixir of life."

Health screenings, such as a baseline test for bone density at menopause can early alert younger women to beginning bone loss. Such tests are now approved by the FDA, their results exact and dependable.

In addition to calcium supplements, experimental studies for osteoporosis, mostly done in the latter part of this decade, have been reported by two researchers at the University of California Medical School at San Francisco. Dr. Steven Harris, Professor of Medicine, radiologist, and Dr. Harry Genant, radiologist, found that Etridonate blocks mineral loss. The studies done at U.C.S.F used the drug "Didronate," by Proctor and Gamble Pharmaceuticals. Doctors in seven medical centers gave small doses of Didronate plus calcium supplements to 423 women and found that it increased bone density in the spine by 5% and about 2% in hip bones. The rate of fractures of the spine in treated women was reduced by nearly half. This fact alone makes Didronate exciting to this writer; but the really good news is that after 4 years, the side effects associated with estrogen replacement therapy (usually used as an osteoporosis preventative) with Didronate have not appeared.

Other research facilities have been at work on the problems as well, so that now there are more options in medication. See your doctor. He/she has answers.

Many women are wary of estrogens, especially equine (horse) based estrogens. (Some estrogen products are derived from the urine of pregnant mares [female horses]). If you are one of the wary ones, for whatever reason, honor your feelings. Your feelings are extremely important in any basic medical decision.

Your brain can help you sort them out and then deal with them, so that ultimately, you make the right decision.

In my opinion, men tend to resist listening to women's feelings and this includes some busy, self-involved male physicians.

Be a wise medical consumer. Explore your options. Study them well. Then make your decision in cooperation with your caregiver. There are FDA-approved medications available for the treatment of osteoporosis for both men and women—Alendronate (Fosamax) Calcitronin and for women, Premarin. These medications slow and also reverse bone loss. Equally important however is to make sure that you are getting adequate levels of calcium and Vitamin D in your body and to get regular, weight-bearing exercise in order to build bone and keep what bone you have.

So celebrate your options! They are new and shiny. And they did not exist five years ago. Expect real change if women become informed. And I'm beginning to think they will: Hillary Clinton and Tipper Gore have been on the local TV stations urging women to have bone density screenings.

Options are now in place to free women from osteoporosis, its disabling and deadly broken hips and posture-distorting dowager's hump. Or its incredibly shrinking women, whose spines have shortened, leaving them inches shorter than they were in early maturity.

NOTES: Good news is on the near horizon for women's health. Recent medical school entrance classes now have over 50% women (1999)

Risk Factors for Osteoporosis

1. Small, thin frame, Asian or Anglo race.
2. Family history includes osteoporosis.
3. Past menopause.
4. Early or surgically induced menopause.
5. High thyroid medication dosage or cortisone-type drugs used for asthma, arthritis, cancer.
6. Low calcium intake in diet (low dairy products. leafy greens, yogurt).
7. Inactive physically.
8. Excessive cigarette or alcohol use.

CHAPTER 6

Heart Disease

The term Heart Disease is a misnomer. It is a disease of the arteries that causes heart problems-arteries plugged by fat deposits that deprive the heart, a muscle, of oxygen. It is this oxygen deprivation that causes angina. Arterial clogging, part of the aging process, starts in childhood.

As in all disease, lifestyle has an impact. Not surprisingly the incidence of heart disease is lower in less-industrialized societies. Inactivity and diet are involved with arterial disease also. Unrelieved stress is believed by many researches to contribute to higher incidence. The jury is still out on this question.

High blood pressure adds to heart disease risk. Exercise is advised because it lowers blood pressure by activating muscles: muscles have an abundance of capillaries and if blood can escape into hundreds and hundreds of capillaries, pressure is reduced.

As for stress and heart disease, Dr. Redford Williams of Duke University has studied the effect of hostile feelings on the heart and has found that angry people have more heart disease than peaceful ones. He has also found in clinical studies that relaxation training when combined with psychological support slows the progress of heart disease.

Dr. Williams is professor of psychology and director of the Behavioral Medical Research Center at Duke University, Durham, North Carolina.

Dr. Dean Ornish, a well-known healer and researcher in the field, has discovered in his research that "early as 1900, two thirds of the protein in the typical American diet came from plant foods, whereas today two thirds of our protein comes from animal foods." Numerous studies have shown that a diet low in animal products lowers the risk levels of heart disease. The Framingham, Massachusetts Heart Study is the one cited most often in this regard.

Older women particularly should be aware that their risk of heart disease quadruples after menopause, when protection afforded by estrogen hormones ends. Women at midlife and beyond should take a grass roots approach to their health—on their own reduce stress, make a real effort to stop smoking, learn yoga (or do other exercise they enjoy) and cut excess fat from the diet. Above all, they should avoid like poison what has been called an epidemic of inactivity; and firmly keep in mind that adding more than five pounds to their frame after age 21 can add to their health risks in many ways.

REFLECTIONS ON HEART DISEASE

To live in our time and witness people self-destruct-die far too early or be victimized by chronic illness as a direct result of unwise lifestyle choices, is to wonder why, if you are a thoughtful person. Social problems are human problems, compounded. Certainly one fruitful way to look at this problem is to try to see the human pain behind the statistics. Pain is part of life and so is our humanity if we value a life of wholeness.

Some years ago psychiatrist David Riesman, M.D. wrote a book called *The Lonely Crowd.* It was an exploration of the causes of disconnection and loneliness in modern society. In some ways since then, we have evolved from loneliness to alienation, despair or isolation, all states that take a deadly toll on mental, spiritual and physical health for most people.

There does exist a small minority of people who prefer to be alone and who do it well at it. I personally have known several such people. And, of course, health researchers report that the healthiest people in the U.S.A. are unmarried, older women. Men are thought to be more isolated than women, single or married, probably because men's lives are not bound up so much with people concerns. Andrew Wiel, author of the best seller *You Can Heal Yourself,* has noted that our relationships with others do affect our over-all health.

The pain of loneliness and isolation leads some of us to unwise lifestyle choices. Dean Ornish quotes food writer B who says, "Fat coats my nerves and numbs the pain." One way or another, people must deal with pain. Our society likes a speedy fix for pain—witness the TV ads, etc.—the speedier, the better. And this is not just a modern approach—it has been around in American culture for a long, long time.

Every single one of us is vulnerable to bad choices. And every single one of us has made a bad decision at some point in our lives. Those of us who have escaped dire consequences of such decisions have no call to be self-righteous, in this writer's opinion.

In this country, choices and opinions are all open to all of us. One can make new choices at any time. Big changes are easier than small changes according to Dr. Dean Ornish. He has found with his heart patients that the payoff to a big change is so evident to the person in his program (which are Spartan, but which work) that such change is nearly always an awesome experience. Truly life changing. I have also personally known several people whose lives were transformed by yoga; I am one of those people.

Indeed, I have been a close friend of a beautiful lady who found in yoga an answer to a long-standing drug problem. She became part of a yoga community, practiced and taught successfully for four or five years and then fell back into the drug scene and disappeared.

This is the way human life goes sometimes. And when I think of my young friend, I am glad I was kind to her. Kindness helps build community.

And our country desperately needs a community spirit, now, as we head into an exciting new century. A spirit and community that includes all ages.

Our current history is calling us to closer ties with our own country men/women and with the world.

Let's listen....

CHAPTER 7

Overweight

This is not a weight-loss book but a few ideas gleaned from years of reading on nutrition and talking to nutritionists, plus too much personal experience with the Over Forty Weight Syndrome may be worthwhile.

The best advice on overweight that I could give would be GET UP AND MOVE, AMERICA!

Balance: a mix of activity and proper eating is the basis of health for everyone. The effects of inactivity and over-eating are devastating after age 40. A fatty diet and a lazy attitude are express tickets to health problems. Excessive alcohol adds a further deadly element; so does cigarette smoking.

As with the rest of the human body, the stomach has its own wisdom, if we will but listen. Ages ago the ancient Egyptians believed that the solar plexus was the seat of the powerful sun god, Ra. Today, millennia later, human inertia and doubt cloud our reasoning and innate good sense about those sacred, miraculous vessels, our bodies.

Awareness of options and of potential problems is critical in older people.

The power in us to change our lives for the better sputters and dies unless recharged by use.

The unfortunate fact is that as we age we do not metabolize fat (or anything else) as efficiently as we did at age 30 or 40. I call this the "fat gap." In simple terms, aging humans do not burn up energy as well as younger ones. Dietary fat is converted to body fat far more easily than carbohydrate and protein because fat already is in a form that can be stored in the cells of the body. When you joke that the waiter's offering, the gorgeous 540 calorie piece of chocolate cake (ganache, Madame? Monsieur?) with thick chocolate frosting goes in your mouth and then right on your hips, your folk wisdom is correct. It does! And unlike fat, it takes work (using up calories) to convert carbohydrates and protein into body fat. The bottom line is calories, however, if you eat too much protein or carbohydrates and don't work it off, it, too, is stored as fat. In addition to the fat gap the liver shrinks in size with age, which makes alcohol metabolism difficult. In women, alcohol is metabolized slower than men at any age. Alcohol contains lots of empty calories. An empty calorie is one that contains zero nourishment. I am not condemning alcohol—the grape is one of God's gifts and moderation is the key.

Since estimates range that from 35 to 60% of American adults are overweight (and a look around your community, no matter where you live, from Alaska to Yuba City to Zanesville, will confirm the statistics) the demographic facts tell us that the battle for normal weight is stalemated. A common sense, easily remembered prescription for health maintenance after age 40 would be to cut calories to 3/4 of what you ate at 30 or 35 years of age; and start exercising.

Try not to back away in horror from these facts. I realize you are human, but this is reality under discussion—the reality of your quality of life for years to come. Do you want to pamper yourself now or do you want seriously to manage your own life? Manage your health? It takes guts and it takes responsible, on-going, motivated structure in your life to accomplish these goals.

Awareness of options and potential problems is excruciatingly important for the elder population. It is folly to discuss cutting calories, without recognizing human food cravings and what to do about them, in my opinion.

I don't know about you, but just the mental picture of a pat of fresh butter on a crunchy roll, or a spoonful of Dreyer's French Vanilla ice cream makes me roll my eyes in pangs of desire. Notice that both of these foods deliver a healthy fat punch.

I'm just about convinced from my own experience with fat cravings over a 25-30 year period, that fat is addictive in some obscure way, its origins either buried in primitive human experience with starvation and semi-starvation; or from body pleasure centers connecting stomach, solar plexus and brain, whatever they may be.

We know from scientific research that human need for fat in the diet was established early in history in prehistoric times to help protect the species from the elements and the risky environment. As back-up in periods when food was scarce, fat was stored as a survival aid. When we overindulge our cravings for fat, it is that ancient ancestor that is calling to us.

Think about it! Are you a cave man or cave woman? No? Then you surely do need some fat in your diet to stay well, but probably nowhere near the amount that you presently consume.

Stroke is a genetic factor in my maternal family and I know that cutting fat is a helpful practice for me. So the battle I have waged over time (while eye-ing the mayonnaise with great longing at times) is guided by this negative health factor. A healthy vanity is certainly in the mix, as everyone feels better when looking fit. I also feel better on a low-fat, moderate calorie diet—"lighter," if you will. The difference is subtle but real.

Resist fattening foods in the following ways:

1. Drink a glass (or probably two) of water. Research at the University of Michigan has proven that two glasses of water (no calories) are more satiating than a can of cola (160 calories). Volume counts (for at least the first hour) in quelling a food crave. Drink water not only to control food craves, but ideally six or seven glasses a day. This curbs appetite and snacking. Water is a food which brings balance to the body chemistry, is as important as food for health.

2. Don't start a diet and exercise plan at the same time. According to professional dietician Patricia Bergen, this combination can lead to fatigue. Start the exercise program first, then, when metabolism is upped a little and your system and your life are adjusted, start the diet.

3. Try to eliminate mindless snacking. Keep tempting foods out of the house or at least out of sight.

4. Avoid fat and alcohol as much as possible. One half a glass of wine satisfies.

5. Distract yourself......by doing something that truly absorbs you when an urge to eat takes over. The urge may go away.

6. Try to convince yourself that healthy eating and competent self-care are more involved in weight maintenance than is will power.

In truth, will power is not the key to health, common sense and self love are. When the Golden Rule says "love your neighbor as yourself" it is not a call to narcissism—it is a call to care....for ourselves and others.

Women crave chocolate more than any other food. (Men are not immune). Fight chocolate cravings with super quality chocolate in small amounts. Two small squares of Cadbury English Milk Chocolate satisfies. Low-cal hot chocolate is another goody. Mini-Tootsie Rolls are a help. No less an authority than Johns Hopkins University has found that an apple or an orange will not satisfy a chocolate crave.

My health idol, Charles Horn, chided the yoga class he taught, "Americans eat too much! You don't need all that food." He strongly recommended fasting one day a week, taking only diluted juice or water. This class of educated people groaned loudly in response to these suggestions.

What we eat, like much of our daily lives is largely a matter of habit. Food cravings fit in this category. Nutritionists have found, interestingly enough, that it's a bad idea to try to banish our food favorites from our daily diet. This usually leads to rebound eating. (We load up more than ever on our favorites because we feel deprived.) Common sense also argues that this would be a bad idea psychologically. In yet another direction, research shows that people maintaining a low-fat diet for as short a term as three months learn to crave the foods on the low-fat diet. The message is that you can change your food cravings. As always, awareness helps; so does information.

Let's insert a bit of philosophy into all of this food talk. The way we look at our bodies and at new ideas about them is the result of both culture and biology. The integration of body and mind is a scary outrageous idea to many people in Western culture. And yet to be a whole person, at home in one's body, mind and spirit (or "soul"—our essence) is desired by many. A person uncomfortable in his/her body finds such a goal difficult to pursue. Many Americans are uncomfortable in their bodies or view the body mechanistically.

Paradoxically, many Americans also have an ongoing desire for such a goal as integration of the whole person (peace or wholeness): How else explain the early best sellerdom of Thomas Merton's works as well as the recent eyebrow-raising volume sales of Thomas Moore's Care of the Soul and his newer book Soulmates. Still other such books are the works of Scott Peck; Bill Moyers; Joan Borysenko-all consistent heavy sellers.

Sales of these books imply a longing for change and exploration into a deeper life. Yoga leads in that direction. It acquaints (or re-acquaints) you with your body, bolsters your mind and spirit, heals the ancient rift.

C. Everett Koop, MD, former Surgeon General of the United States, kicked off the first official national campaign against overweight a few years ago with a national television broadcast on prime time.

As one of the most effective Surgeon Generals in US history, his slogan "Shape Up America" tackles the problem of overweight and obesity, the biggest cause of preventable illness and death in this country. His ideas echo the ideas in this chapter.

Figures released three years ago by Dr. Koop indicated 35% of all adult women and 31% of all American men were obese.

Figures recently released by the National Heart, Lung & Blood Institute, National Institutes of Health reported the latest information:

59.4% of men in the U.S. are overweight or obese.

50.7% of women in the U.S. are overweight or obese.

Staggering! Obesity is dramatically increasing the risk of heart disease, high blood pressure and diabetes.

Dr. Koop has stated the sad fact that the medical community has been sitting on the sidelines while the disease of obesity has mushroomed into a public crisis. He summed it up by requesting doctors to measure body mass index and appealing to the American public to eat less and exercise more.

As part of a sound health program, yoga can play a major role in Koop's preventative campaign. We are delighted he has exerted his formidable stature to fight obesity and overweight.

Determine your own weight report card according to Metropolitan Life Insurance Company's height and weight tables on the next page.

If you weigh too much, remember Dr. Koop's advice; EAT LESS AND EXERCISE MORE.

If your weight is right on or close, Bravo!

Table 10. 1983 Metropolitan Life Insurance Co.
height and weight tables (21)

height	small frame	medium frame	large frame
	◄──────────────lbs──────────────►		
men*			
5' 2"	128-134	131-141	138-150
5' 3"	130-136	133-143	140-153
5' 4"	132-138	135-145	142-156
5' 5"	134-140	137-148	144-160
5' 6"	136-142	139-151	146-164
5' 7"	138-145	142-154	149-168
5' 8"	140-148	145-157	152-172
5' 9"	142-151	148-160	155-176
5' 10"	144-154	151-163	158-180
5' 11"	146-157	154-166	161-184
6' 0"	149-160	157-170	164-188
6' 1"	152-164	160-174	168-192
6' 2"	155-168	164-178	172-197
6' 3"	158-172	167-182	176-202
6' 4"	162-176	171-187	181-207
women‡			
4' 10"	102-111	109-121	118-131
4' 11"	103-113	111-123	120-134
5' 0"	104-115	113-126	122-137
5' 1"	106-118	115-129	125-140
5' 2"	108-121	118-132	128-143
5' 3"	111-124	121-135	131-147
5' 4"	114-127	124-138	134-151
5' 5"	117-130	127-141	137-155
5' 6"	120-133	130-144	140-159
5' 7"	123-136	133-147	143-163
5' 8"	126-139	136-150	146-167
5' 9"	129-142	139-153	149-170
5' 10"	132-145	142-156	152-173
5' 11"	135-148	145-159	155-17h
6' 0"	138-151	148-162	158-179

*Weights at ages 25–59 based on lowest mortality. Weight in pounds according to frames (in indoor clothing weighing 5 lbs., shoes with 1" heels).
‡Weights at ages 25–59 based on lowest mortality. Weight in pounds according to frames (in indoor clothing weighing 3 lbs., shoes with 1" heels).
Courtesy of Metropolitan Life Insurance Company, Statistical Bulletin.

Part 2

YOGA AND WELL BEING

CHAPTER 8

Nutrition

Would it surprise you to learn that 82% of adults interviewed via telephone survey for a recent nutrition test flunked the test or got a D grade? Or that participants reported they read labels, but the test showed that they could not apply label information as a practical matter to get a baseline healthy diet?

The survey also revealed that a major trap on the path to healthier eating habits is the fear of having to bypass favorite foods. This amazing fact unearthed by scientific study will not come as a surprise to most of us. Unmasked again!

As for the professional nutrition community, it was faulted for causing public confusion by releasing information that contradicts previous nutritional advice, while failing to explain such actions.

A subsequent survey of supermarket shoppers published in the Wall Street Journal, showed that in American supermarkets, 8.9 percent more money is spent on carbonated soft drinks than on milk. Cigarettes and beer are supermarket's biggest revenue producers, which tells us something about lifestyle choices. Ice cream, cookies and candy all rank among the top twenty.

Meat consumption has been dropping, which might mean healthier diet, but the same is true of vegetables. The Chicago firm responsible for these statistics, the N.P.D. Group, has tracked eating habits nationwide since 1982. The Group's vice president, Harry Balzer, noted that only 29.32 per cent of home-prepared meals included vegetables (potatoes excluded) during the latest time-track of one year. This is the lowest vegetable consumption figure since the tracking started, in 1981.

Fruit and vegetable consumption is of concern because over the last decade, scientific evidence has grown that boosting the fruit and vegetable intake in the population lowers disease risk, including lung, prostate, bladder, esophagus and stomach cancers.

Science does not know yet what element in fruits and vegetables is the protective one. However, the evidence is heavy that such a protective factor exists. Until it is isolated, the best course is to eat a wide variety of these foods. California nutritionists in 1992 recommended five servings a day, and this advisory since has been adopted nationwide in the profession. Six ounces of juice or 1/2 cup of solid constitutes a serving of fruits and vegetables. In addition to their other valuable characteristics, these foods are fat-free healthy snacks for those who are overweight.

The one healthy food category that did advance in the survey noted above was cereal, which placed third in supermarket revenues. (Whether increased dollar volume reflects the huge cereal price increases over the past few years is not known.) The survey reported that shoppers do sense that cereal is a healthy food. Professional dieticians report that fiber lowers fats and sugars in the blood and prevents constipation, a real problem for many inactive older adults. The professional dietician I consulted about fiber, Peggy Morrow, R.D. of San Jose, California, recommends thinking of fiber in simple terms, whole grain bread or cereals, fruits and vegetables, legumes such as lentils and beans will suffice.

As long as we eat, nutrition will be with us. But food should be a friend, not an anxiety-producer as it is to many Americans today. To use current terms, they obsess about it. Comforting words on the subject came recently from Dr. Walter Mertz, one-time chair of the Council on Nutrition, U.S. Department of Agriculture. In a speech to the Council he gave three basic nutrition guidelines:

Eat a varied diet. He speaks admiringly of the Japanese diet, which tries to incorporate 31 different foodstuffs in a day.

Enjoy your food!

For insurance, a multiple vitamin tablet a day. What could be simpler?

Some medical doctors also recommend that older adults add to the multiple vitamin tablet, 400mg of Vitamin E (thought to protect against heart attack) plus 1,000mg Vitamin C to aid immunity (the immune system flags in its daily miracles as humans age.)

Carol Ceresa, MHSL, Registered Dietitian, Chief, Clinical Nutrition, Veterans Administration Medical Center, San Francisco, cautions "Before you put anything in your body, either a supplement or a food, give it careful consideration and don't take any nutritional claim at face value. It could result in negative health consequences and needless monetary drain." Ms. Ceresa adds that "What food provides cannot be packaged in a pill." There is no joy in pill-taking. Food should be a source of pleasure to us.

There is inconsistency in nutritional reporting. For this reason, Dr. Mertz' advice noted above, is excellent and is reassuring in its simplicity and common sense appeal.

Nutrition, Target Weight

Self observation of personal food habits is crucial. In time, for example, through such observation, I found that a consistent, one glass of wine for me, seven days a week, would add 2 lbs. within 2 weeks. At first I could not believe it. I then decided to try just having wine on week-ends—Friday night, Saturday and Sunday. This method worked! I had my wine and did not gain weight.

So evolved my week-end diet, or never on Friday after 5 pm, Saturday or Sunday. I still use this method when I find my weight creeping up. I eat what I want on week-ends, have my glass or 1/2 glass of wine then, too, and as the 20-somethings in the family say, 'No Problema!' Bear in mind that you cannot go wild and binge on week- ends; sedate behavior is called for. Even with that small caveat, the program certainly beats the deprivation factor experienced on the all week, every day of the week diet for me. Best of all, it works!

Getting to basics, how much fat is too much fat? Here is a formula that is helpful. It comes from Jim Wood former food columnist of the San Francisco Examiner, a man who savors his food and wine but still looks very much in line as far as weight. Below is the fat formula according to Jim Wood: (You'll need pencil and paper.)

First, write down your present weight. Multiply it by 13 if you are a moderately active person, a little more if you're very active (15 would be a good number), and 12 if you're an admitted couch potato or relatively inactive.

Divide the answer by 5, and the total will be the number of fat calories that are o.k. for you to consume each day. The figure is on the low side of accepted levels of fat consumption, but that's where we're healthiest. This fat figuring can be tricky, since fat totals are sometimes stated in grams instead of calories. In that case, simply multiply the number of grams by nine—e.g., 9 grams of fat, 90 calories.

Wood's formula can also work as a diet. Use your target weight rather than your real weight as the multiplier number. Jim Wood says that using this formula with his desired weight (target weight) for the multiplier number, he is able to lose a pound a week. He calls the method "painless." In my thinking, no weight loss method is painless. On those occasions when I want marble fudge ice cream and can't have it, I agree with Jesse "Big Daddy" Unruh (he earned the title) who, when asked by a reporter how he had taken off multiple tens of pounds and kept it off, opined, "Basically, I don't eat anything I like." Unruh was for years Speaker of the House, California State Legislature. Most of the time I try to be realistic about eats, as Jesse was in his own way.

Planning consciously your day or week of eating nourishing food is a great start on facing reality about food and you. Planning is important, but no plan works without commitment. Commitment is key for changing long embedded habits.

And remember, BE KIND TO YOURSELF.

Nutrition, How to Hold a Target Weight Once You Have Achieved It Eating, Pleasure or Battle?

Nothing in life is constant except change. You can change! Commitment is your primary tool for changing life-long habits, including eating habits. You can change from Battleground Eating (perhaps a remnant of childhood?) to Power Eating, eating that puts you in control and does good things for you and your physical and emotional self. Spending your days thinking only of what you can't eat and then soon or late, eating in conflict, is a no-win lifestyle. It's a prescription for misery, for we all must eat. Why be miserable when a bit of planning (a mature way to think) will eliminate it?

Some time ago, I was in a situation with food that seemed to have no way out. No matter how closely I monitored what I ate, I kept gaining weight. I was extremely active physically, and yet I seemed to have nowhere to go but up on the scale.

Serendipity came to the rescue: I was in a Doctor's office on another matter and I had noticed before that this particular man was trim-looking and did not look deprived. So I asked him, "What's your secret for staying trim?" "I weigh every day," was his answer, "And if I've gained a couple of ounces or more over my target weight, I cut back on some food that day."

'Talk about the Zen of weight loss!' I said to myself. 'This man is not only in the present, he's living it.' And I've been following his rule ever since. I have great news: IT WORKS.

A couple of must-do's:
Weigh in the morning, stomach empty. (Water is ok, so is diluted juice.)
Weigh nude.

If you are near your target weight try this first method. I found that with the weigh-every-day method, self observation of personal food habits comes built-in—and pays off handsomely. The entire process of weight stabilization also becomes more matter-of-fact, less emotion-loaded. At least it seemed more matter-of-fact to me, just the facts on the scale, robbed of self-recrimination, calories and a load of emotional baggage. Try to be kind to yourself, as much as possible. The world is not kind, so we must try to be kind to ourselves, and encouraging to the inner person who is trying, trying to maintain a healthful weight.

Healthy Snacks

Snacking is a way of life for most Americans. Delicious, healthful low-calorie foods are available; choose your snacks wisely, keeping over-all food goals in mind. Here are some healthy snacks that stave off hunger at 10:30 am, 3 or 4 pm.

2 tsp. of peanut butter, neat, is a real winner. (50 calories.) Halts hunger pangs for at least an hour.
Good Earth tea, which has a rich, satisfying herbal-spice flavor and a heavenly aroma, is also a great diet help between meals. Comes caffeinated and decaffeinated. The caffeinated blend is extremely satisfying, almost making you forget about food; and while the decaf is less so, for this purpose it's delicious and it works.

Here is a yummy list, all low calorie.
1 hard cooked egg–50 calories
1-1/2 cup light popcorn–70 calories

1 cup raw mushrooms–25 calories (dust with Mexican seasoning)

1 medium carrot–25 calories

1 small tomato–25 calories

15 radishes–25 calories

1/2 cup low fat cottage cheese–50 calories

3 stalks celery–25 calories (pave these with cottage cheese—yum!)

1/2 banana–40 calories

1/2 apple–40 calories

1/2 grapefruit–40 calories

1 slice chewy whole grain bread, with preserves (modest)–70 calories

3/4 c. papaya–40 calories

12 grapes–40 calories

1 cup watermelon–40 calories

3/4 c. cucumber–25 calories (sprinkle with good vinegar and a wisp of sugar, French style)

6 ounces tomato juice–40 calories

1 peach (medium)–40 calories

2/3 c. plain yogurt (low fat)–70 calories

Rye crisp (2)–70 calories

1/2 white or sweet potato, yam–70 calories

1 medium tangerine–40 calories

Oyster crackers (20)–70 calories

3 low-fat graham crackers–75 calories

6 saltines–70 calories

1/3 c. rice–70 calories

Crispix (2/3 c.)–70 calories (no milk)

Shredded Wheat–(3/4 biscuit + 1/3 c. milk) 85 calories

Weetabix (1 biscuit + 1/3 c. milk)–70 calories

For an easy, filling soup, mini-caloried but scrumptious, combine tomato juice or V-8 and cooked rice (2 c. juice, 1/3 c. rice + bay leaf or parsley. Simmer a few minutes (4 or 5) or pop in microwave. Add 1/2 tsp butter to your cup when you serve it.) Sip and enjoy!

I would save cheese, frozen yogurt, granola bars, candy, cookies, ice cream and nuts for dessert on weekends. Potato chips are a real week-end treat, too.

Good Words About Eating, Plus Menus by Peggy Morrow Dietician, Graduate U.C. Davis

These menus can be individualized with appropriate substitutions such as:

1. Alcoholic Beverages—Zero to 1 to 2 servings, 1 to 2 times per week.

2. Eggs—Substitute with egg substitute product or use real eggs minus yolks.

3. Dressings & Fats—Use low or no fat dressings, mayonnaise, sour cream (all readily available at food markets); margarine.

4. Beverages—Herbal teas, decaffeinated coffees, bottled water, juices.

5. Dairy Foods—Use non, low-fat or regular milk. Low-fat cottage cheese, soy based cheeses; non-fat, low-fat, or regular yogurts; ice milk, sorbets, sherbets, etc.

6. Breads & Cereals—Use whole grain breads, bran-type cereals, granolas, low-fat crackers, rice cakes.

7. Always take advantage of seasonal fruits and vegetables. Including a variety ensures best nutrient intake. Be adventurous and try new ones or new ways to prepare them.

8. Snacks between meals and before bedtime are optional; individual caloric needs should be considered.

9. Do not deny yourself treats occasionally so as to avoid "bingeing" on a particular food.

Food and meals are to be enjoyed.

Peggy Morrow's Menus

	Day 1	Day 2	Day 3	Day 4	Day 5
	Cantaloupe	Juice	1/2 Banana	Raisins in	Fruit
	Bran Cereal	Peanut Butter on	Falafel Eggs	Hot Cereal	Fried Rice with
	Non-fat Milk	Toast	Toasts	1/2 English Muffin	Egg & Peas
	Tea/Coffee	Tea/Coffee	Tea/Coffee	Juice/Coffee	Tea/Juice
	Yogurt - 1 cup	Tofu Cheese	Tuna Sandwich	Humus	Yogurt - 1 cup
	1/2 Sandwich	Crackers	Coleslaw	Pocket Bread	Rice Cakes
	(Turkey)	Carrot Sticks	Cup Vegetable Soup	Lettuce/Tomato/	Bowl Cream Soup
	Fruit	Grapes	Milk/Water	Cucumber	Juice/Milk
	Water/Juice	Water/Milk		Fruit	
				Milk/Juice	
	Beef Frank (kabobs)	Baked Chicken	Caesar Salad	Broiled Catfish	Lasagne
	Rice	(skinless)	French Bread	Rice Pilaf	Tossed Salad with
	Stir Fried Vegetables	Potato Torte	Kiwis	Steamed Vegetables	Dressing
	Water/Milk/Wine	Salad with Dressing	Milk/Juice	Water/Milk/Juice	Sourdough Bread
		Juice/Milk/Water	Tapioca Pudding	String Beans	

Menus

Day 6	Day 7	Day 8	Day 9	Day 10
Juice	Juice	Fruit	Juice	1/2 Banana
Vegetable Omelette	1/2 Banana	Cheese/Grn. Onion	French Toast	Bagel with Non-fat
Toast	Granola	Melted on Tortilla	Maple Syrup	Cream Cheese & Lox
Coffee/Milk/Tea	Milk	Milk/Coffee	2 Sausages	Milk
	Coffee/Tea		Milk	Coffee/Tea
			Coffee/Milk	
Bowl Beef Noodle Soup	Curried Shrimp	Cream of Potato Soup	Chinese Chicken Salad	Pasta Salad with
Crackers	Garbanzo Bean Salad	Sesame Roll	2 Spring Rolls	Low-fat Salame
Fruit	Rice Cakes	1/2 Roast Beef Sand.	Tea/Juice	Crackers
Juice/Milk	Vegetable Relishes	Grapes	2 Fortune Cookies	Fruit/Apple
	Juice/Tea	Milk/Tea/Juice	Milk/Juice/Water	Milk/Juice/Water
Meatloaf	Turkey Casserole with Pasta	Bean/Sausage Casserole	Eggplant Parmesan	Roast Pork Tenderloin
Mashed Potatoes	Wheat Dinner Rolls	Corn Bread	Bread Sticks	Applesauce
Gravy	Sauteed Snow Peas	Salad with Dressing	Green Salad with Dressing	Twice Baked Potatoes
Steamed Vegetables	Milk/Water	Juice/Water/Milk	Milk/Juice/Water	Squash - Yellow
Water/Juice/Milk	2 Cookies			Milk/Water/Tea

Menus

Day 11	Day 12	Day 13	Day 14
Juice	Melon/Berries	Juice	Juice
Olive-Avocado-	Pancakes	Hot Cereal	Poached Egg
Cheese Omelette	Maple Syrup	Toast - Raisin Bread	Toast
Toast	Bacon	Milk	Milk
Milk/Coffee/Tea	Milk/Coffee/Tea	Coffee/Tea	Coffee/Tea
2 Vegetarian	Baked Potato with	Grilled Hamburger	Minestrone Soup
Pizza Slices	Chile Beans/Cheese	lettuce/tomato	Rustic Bread
Fruit	Squaw Bread	1/2 Order Fries	Kalamata Olive Spread
Tea/Juice/Milk	Fruit - orange	Juice/Tea/Milk	Fruit
Brownie	Tea/Milk/Water	Fruit (Pineapple)	Milk/Juice/Water
Grilled Red Snapper	Spaghetti with	Cheese Enchiladas	Teriyaki Chicken
Couscous	Meatballs	Mexican Style Rice	Rice
Steamed Veggies	French Bread	Boiled Pinto Beans	Napa Cabbage
Juice/Milk/Tea	Tossed Green Salad	Sliced Tomatoes	Pickled Carrots & Daikon
	with Dressing	Beer/Water/Tea	Tea/Water/Juice
	Milk/Tea/Water	Flan	
	Sorbet		

The Traditional Healthy Mediterranean Diet Pyramid

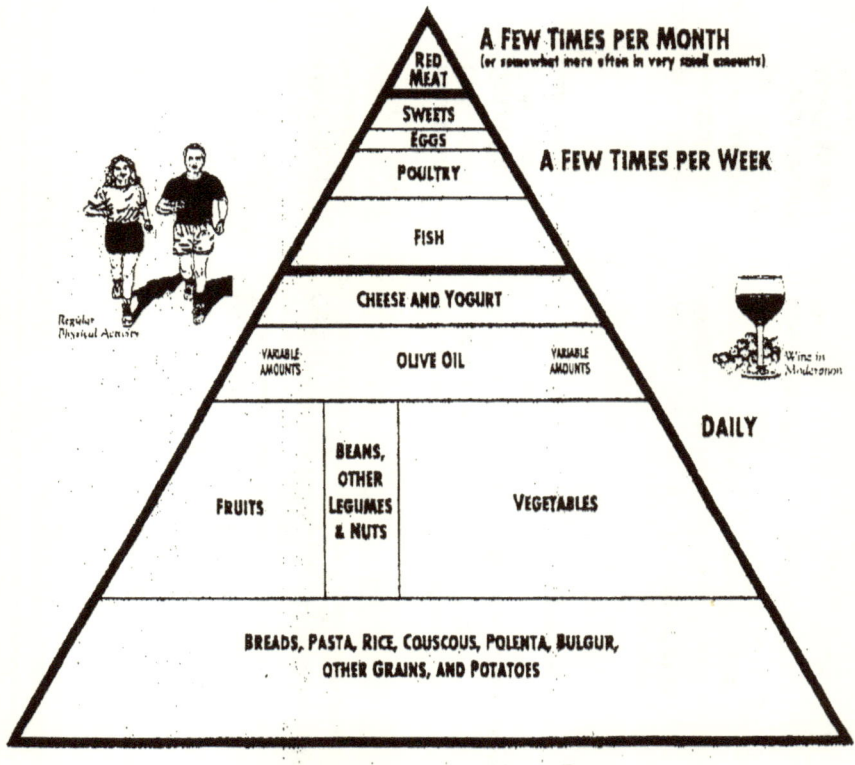

A FEW TIMES PER MONTH
(or somewhat more often in very small amounts)

RED MEAT

SWEETS

EGGS

POULTRY

A FEW TIMES PER WEEK

FISH

CHEESE AND YOGURT

Regular Physical Activity

VARIABLE AMOUNTS   OLIVE OIL   VARIABLE AMOUNTS

Wine in Moderation

FRUITS

BEANS, OTHER LEGUMES & NUTS

VEGETABLES

DAILY

BREADS, PASTA, RICE, COUSCOUS, POLENTA, BULGUR, OTHER GRAINS, AND POTATOES

© Copyright 1994 Oldways Preservation & Exchange Trust

The Traditional Healthy Asian Diet Pyramid

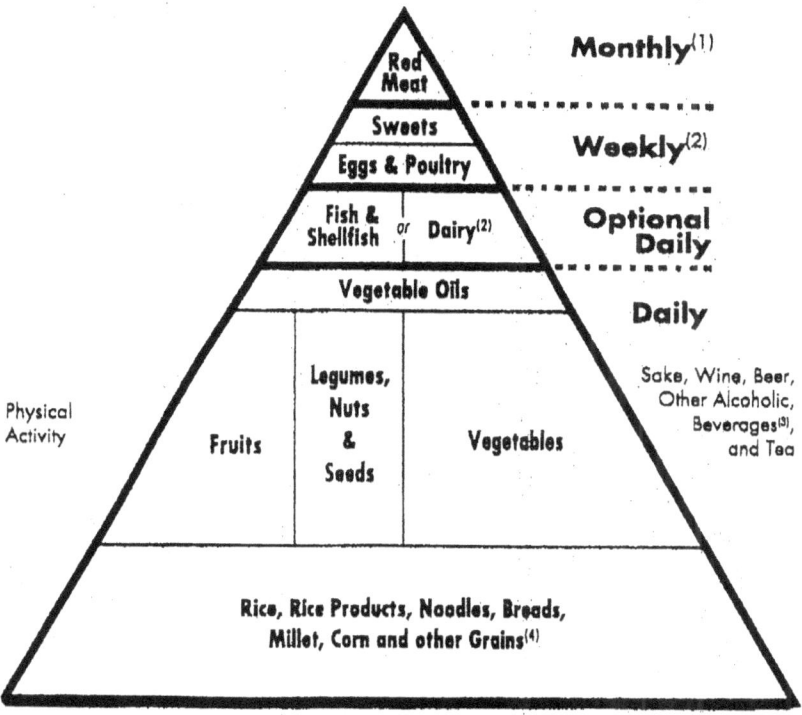

©1995 Oldways Preservation & Exchange Trust

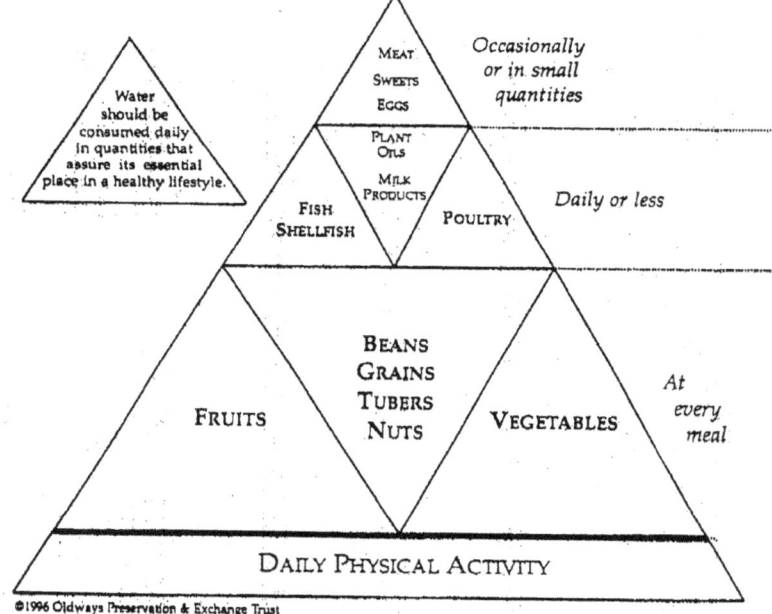

Official Version November 22, 1996

HEALTHY TRADITIONAL LATIN AMERICAN DIET PYRAMID

Preliminary Concept Based on Principles of Healthy Traditional Latin American Diets

This healthy traditional Latin American Diet Pyramid reflects Latin American dietary traditions historically associated with good health. It is one of a group of food guide pyramids developed in a series of conferences — Public Health Implications of Traditional Diets — that consider diverse dietary traditions around the world. These pyramids, a principal objective of the conferences, are intended to stimulate greater dialogue and interest in cultural models for healthy eating. This Latin American Diet Pyramid is considered preliminary and subject to revision in light of ongoing nutrition research.

Water should be consumed daily in quantities that assure its essential place in a healthy lifestyle.

MEAT
SWEETS
EGGS

Occasionally or in small quantities

PLANT OILS

MILK PRODUCTS

FISH SHELLFISH   POULTRY

Daily or less

BEANS
GRAINS
TUBERS
NUTS

FRUITS   VEGETABLES

At every meal

DAILY PHYSICAL ACTIVITY

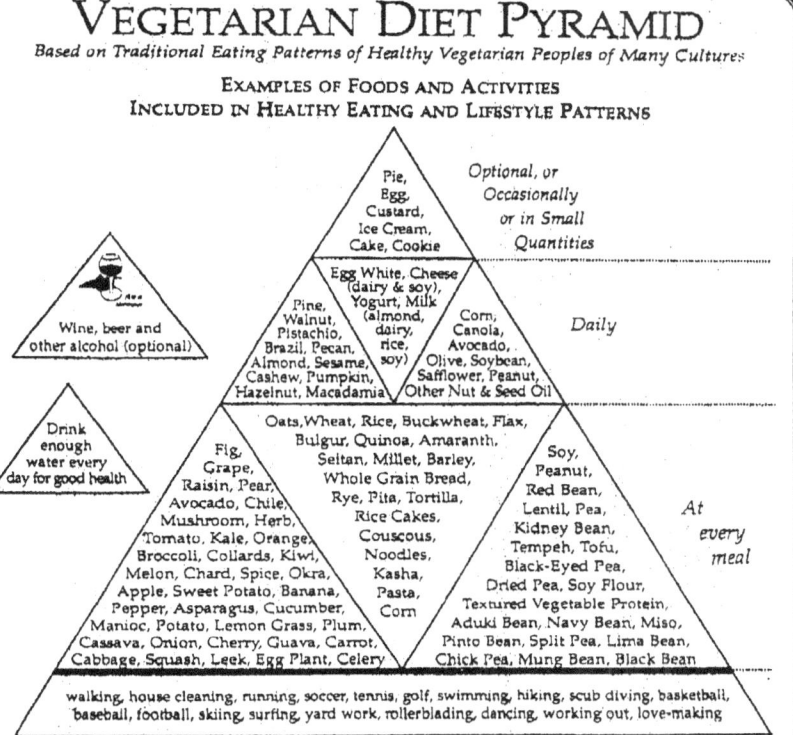

VEGETARIAN DIET PYRAMID

Based on Traditional Eating Patterns of Healthy Vegetarian Peoples of Many Cultures

EXAMPLES OF FOODS AND ACTIVITIES
INCLUDED IN HEALTHY EATING AND LIFESTYLE PATTERNS

Pie, Egg, Custard, Ice Cream, Cake, Cookie — *Optional, or Occasionally or in Small Quantities*

Egg White, Cheese (dairy & soy), Yogurt, Milk (almond, dairy, rice, soy) — Pine, Walnut, Pistachio, Brazil, Pecan, Almond, Sesame, Cashew, Pumpkin, Hazelnut, Macadamia — Corn, Canola, Avocado, Olive, Soybean, Safflower, Peanut, Other Nut & Seed Oil — *Daily*

Wine, beer and other alcohol (optional)

Drink enough water every day for good health

Oats, Wheat, Rice, Buckwheat, Flax, Bulgur, Quinoa, Amaranth, Seitan, Millet, Barley, Whole Grain Bread, Rye, Pita, Tortilla, Rice Cakes, Couscous, Noodles, Kasha, Pasta, Corn — Fig, Grape, Raisin, Pear, Avocado, Chile, Mushroom, Herb, Tomato, Kale, Orange, Broccoli, Collards, Kiwi, Melon, Chard, Spice, Okra, Apple, Sweet Potato, Banana, Pepper, Asparagus, Cucumber, Manioc, Potato, Lemon Grass, Plum, Cassava, Onion, Cherry, Guava, Carrot, Cabbage, Squash, Leek, Egg Plant, Celery — Soy, Peanut, Red Bean, Lentil, Pea, Kidney Bean, Tempeh, Tofu, Black-Eyed Pea, Dried Pea, Soy Flour, Textured Vegetable Protein, Aduki Bean, Navy Bean, Miso, Pinto Bean, Split Pea, Lima Bean, Chick Pea, Mung Bean, Black Bean — *At every meal*

walking, house cleaning, running, soccer, tennis, golf, swimming, hiking, scub diving, basketball, baseball, football, skiing, surfing, yard work, rollerblading, dancing, working out, love-making

CHAPTER 9

The Importance Of The Breath In Yoga

Improved breathing techniques are a vital source of wellness in yoga. Each breath we take brings into the body vital, life-giving oxygen; each breath exhaled is filled with body waste products. Energy-filled fresh oxygen thus is brought to the blood, joints and musculature, invigorating the entire system.

To the yoga student, breath is life. Accordingly, Linda Zecca's breathing instructions follow.

Linda's Breathing Instructions

1. Tuning in to the breath.
2. The complete breath.

Lie on the floor on the back. Have the arms along side the body, palms facing upward. The feet are slightly apart. Begin by relaxing the facial muscles; just tell them to relax and they will relax. Feel the relaxation flow through the neck, through the shoulders and then through the rest of the body.

It is now time to tune in to the breath. Do not consciously change the breath in any way; simply observe the natural inhale and the natural exhale. You can do this by placing the awareness on the chest, feeling as it rises and lowers; or at the nostrils noting as the air comes in and is expelled. Continue to observe the breath for two to three minutes.

Following the last exhale of this round of breathing, begin the complete breath. If you are new to the breath, place your hand on the abdomen. Inhale now and feel the abdomen expand. Have a slight pause and then exhale, feeling the abdomen pull in and contract. Continue for a few rounds. Remember always to include a pause after the inhale and after the exhale. It is said at the pause between the breaths is where real peace and relaxation occur.

After a few rounds, we take the breath a little deeper. Inhale, expand the abdomen and allow the air to rise to the rib cage area. Take in a little more air and bring it to the upper chest area; so as we inhale and the abdomen expands, we bring in the air first to fill the lower lungs, then the mid-lungs, and then the upper lungs. To exhale, reverse the process. Expel the air first from the upper chest area, then the rib cage area and last the abdomen, fully contracting and pulling in the abdomen at the end of the exhale.

The process involved in this breath is similar to filling and emptying a glass of water. First you fill the lower part of the glass, then the middle and then the top. To empty the glass you start from the top, then go to the middle and then the bottom. And so it is with the breath.

Do several minutes of the complete breath at your own pace. Have the breathing slow, deep and relaxed. Place the mental awareness on the breath and aim to keep the awareness here. If the mind wanders, as soon as you notice this, gently bring it back to the breath.

Such gentle attempts to focus upon the breath, with time, bring the gifts of concentration, peace and knowledge of the self.

Take a deep breath of air and fill the lower lungs. Take in a little more air and fill the mid-lungs. Take in a little more air and fill the upper lungs. Now open the mouth and allow the air to come gushing out.

Bring your awareness to your shoulders. Just tell the shoulders to relax and they will relax. Tense up the shoulders. Bring them together as if they were going to meet at a point in the middle of your chest. Squeeze tighter, tighter, tighter and release. Now gently roll your head from right to left and back to center.

Have the eyes closed now and open your mouth and move the jaw around. Now, stick out the tongue and open the mouth and move the jaw around. Now, stick out the tongue and open the mouth as wide as possible, without forcing or straining. Stretch the entire face as if you were giving a silent scream at something. Stretch, stretch and release.

Now make a monkey face. Gently scrunch up the face as if the whole face was meeting at the tip of your nose. Squeeze again.......and release. Now that we have gone over the body, tensing and relaxing the various parts physically, let's go over the body mentally.

Start with the feet. Relax the toes. Just tell the toes to relax, and they will relax. The body obeys the gentle, loving suggestions of the mind. Relax the soles of the feet. Allow the top of the feet to relax. Relax the ankles. Begin to relax the lower legs and the upper legs. Feel the entire leg area relaxing and letting go.

Next bring your attention to the buttocks. Relax the buttocks, relax the pelvic area, relax the hips. Allow the lower back to relax; then the upper back. Begin to relax the rib cage area and the upper chest. Bring your attention to your fingers. Relax the fingers, relax the wrists, relax the hands. Allow the relaxation to flow through the lower arms and the upper arms. Relax the shoulders. Relax the neck.

Begin to relax the facial muscles. Relax the jaw, the chin, the cheeks. Relax the nose, the eyes, the eyelids. Relax the muscles behind the eyes. Relax the temples; relax the forehead. Feel the entire face relaxed. Relax the scalp. Relax the back of the head and the top of the head. As the body relaxes bring your awareness to the mind. If there are any thoughts in the mind, don't get involved with them right now. Watch your thoughts as you would watch leaves floating down a stream. Observe them and let them go.

Next, bring your attention to the breath. Without consciously changing the breath, observe the breath. Observe as you inhale and as you exhale. Get in touch with the natural flow of the breath. Allow yourself to become one with the breath and let the breath take you deeper and deeper into a relaxed, peaceful state. Give yourself three to five minutes of quiet, deep relaxation.

When you have completed this phase, begin to bring the awareness back to the body. Allow the breath to deepen. Take several long deep breaths. Feel as you inhale you are taking new energy in; feel as you exhale you are releasing the old energy out.

Next begin gentle movements in the body: wiggle the toes and fingers. Stretch the arms and legs, slowly. Move the hips and shoulders. Gently rotate the head from side to side. Do whatever feels good to wake the body up.

Now, when you feel ready, roll over to the side, bend the knees, get up and come to a comfortable seated position.

A relaxation suggestion. Most of you own a tape recorder. A good idea is to make a tape of your very own by reading these instructions onto a tape or the parts which you really feel would help.

CHAPTER 10

Deep Relaxation

The relaxation process begins by first tensing then relaxing various parts of the body, continues into ever-deeper body relaxation and then finishes with relaxation of the mind and concentration on the breath, which brings both deep relaxation and a sense of peace, which may be fleeting at first, deepening with practice.

As noted above, begin by tensing then relaxing various body parts. Come to a comfortable lying position on the back. Have the arms along side the body, palms facing upward. Have the feet slightly apart. Begin with the right leg. Stretch the leg out along the floor and then tense it up. Make the muscles really stiff; to do this, point the toe, squeeze leg muscles. Raise the leg off the floor just a bit, two or three inches. Squeeze tighter, tighter...............and release. Allow the leg to fall to the floor, give the ankle a roll and forget about it. Now do the same with the left leg.

Bring your attention next to the right arm. Stretch the arm out and open the fingers really wide. Now begin to tense up the arm; make a tight fist with the hand; make the arm really stiff, as if you were angry with someone. Raise the arm off the floor—just a few inches. Squeeze tighter, tighter, tighter; and release. Let the arm fall to the floor, give the wrist a roll and forget about it. Repeat with the left arm.

Now, bring the attention to the buttock muscles. Tense the muscles up—squeeze the muscles tighter, tighter.........and release.

Take a deep breath of air and fill the lower lungs. Take in a little more air and fill the mid-lungs. Take in a little more air and fill the upper lungs. Now open the mouth and allow the air to come gushing out.

Bring your awareness to your shoulders. Just tell the shoulders to relax and they will relax. Tense up the shoulders. Bring them together as if they were going to meet at a point in the middle of your chest. Squeeze tighter, tighter, tighter...........and release.

Now gently roll your head from right to left and back to center.

Have the eyes closed now and open your mouth and move the jaw around. Now, stick out the tongue and open the mouth and move the jaw around. Now, stick out the tongue and open the mouth as wide as possible, without forcing or straining. Stretch the entire face as if you were giving a silent scream at something. Stretch, stretch..........and release.

Now make a monkey face. Scrunch up the face as if the whole face was meeting at the tip of your nose............... and release.

Now that we have gone over the body, tensing and relaxing the various parts physically, let's go over the body mentally.

Start with the feet. Relax the toes. Just tell the toes to relax, and they will relax. The body obeys the gentle, loving suggestions of the mind. Relax the soles of the feet. Allow the top of the feet to relax. Relax the ankles. Begin to relax the lower legs and the upper legs. Feel the entire leg area relaxing and letting go.

Next bring your attention to the buttocks. Relax the buttocks, relax the pelvic area, relax the hips. Allow the lower back to relax; then the upper back. Begin to relax the rib cage area and the upper chest.

Bring your attention to your fingers. Relax the fingers, relax the wrists, relax the hands. Allow the relaxation to flow through the lower arms and the upper arms. Relax the shoulders. Relax the neck.

Begin to relax the facial muscles. Relax the jaw, the chin, the cheeks. Relax the nose, the eyes, the eyelids. Relax the muscles behind the eyes.

Relax the temples; relax the forehead. Feel the entire face relaxed. Relax the scalp. Relax the back of the head and the top of the head.

As the body relaxes bring your awareness to the mind. If there are any thoughts in the mind, don't get involved with them right now. Watch your thoughts as you would watch leaves floating down a stream. Observe them and let them go.

Next, bring your attention to the breath. Without consciously changing the breath, observe the breath. Observe as you inhale and as you exhale. Get in touch with the natural flow of the breath. Allow yourself to become one with the breath and let the breath take you deeper and deeper into a relaxed, peaceful state.

Give yourself three to five minutes of quiet, deep relaxation.

When you have completed this phase, begin to bring the awareness back to the body. Allow the breath to deepen. Take several long deep breaths. Feel as you inhale you are taking new energy in; feel as you exhale you are releasing the old energy out.

Next begin gentle movements in the body: wiggle the toes and fingers. Stretch the arms and legs, slowly. Move the hips and shoulders. Gently rotate the head from side to side. Do whatever feels good to wake the body up.

Now, when you feel ready, roll over to the right side, bend the knees, get up and come to a comfortable seated position.

A relaxation suggestion. Most of you own a tape recorder. A good idea is to make a tape of your very own by reading these instructions onto a tape or the parts which you really feel would help.

CHAPTER 11

Meditation

Erick Fromm, author and psychiatrist, when asked for a "practical solution to the problems of living" answered, "Quietness. The experience of stillness. You have to stop in order to be able to change directions." Perhaps that is why the sea holds endless fascination for us…A walk on the beach calms, and at a casual glance, the ocean seems a vast, still continent, restful, soothing, while ours is so roiled and hectic.

The practice of meditation can be described as cooling the jets of the mind…cooling the jets so that the brain's neurons stop firing so rapidly and the inner throb of the mind slows. The mind quiet, the innermost person better can be experienced. Meditation is an invitation to be. Your self is in there. Perhaps, a different self–but still one of the facets of you, the person.

You cannot force yourself to relax. It is rather a process of learning and letting go. Your tensions are not outside you; they are inside you. In quietness, the self may find peace, become an integrated whole.

Meditation is a kind of self-directed travel into what Deepak Chopra, M.D. has called "the timeless mind," or spirit, the deep source of strength, relaxation and peace within each of us.

Meditation is about awareness. Awareness, or conscious attention, is the mind's equivalent of physical vision; both have the ability to sharpen or widen our focus. Its roots, 3,000 years old, are in the east, in India,

Tibet. For some, it is the heart of yoga. It is as valid today as when it first was discovered. For many westerners, it works.

As yoga is, meditation is experiential rather than intellectual. That alone makes it challenging to the western person. It is an experiencing of life, rather than a teaching. Benefit comes in the doing, and is cumulative, which speaks of patience.

In 1975, Dr. Herbert Benson of Harvard University wrote a small book, *The Relaxation Response.* In that book, he concluded that the relaxation response is kindred to the flight or fight response, but its physical and neurological opposite. Everyone has felt the rapid breathing, rapid heartbeat and hyper-alertness of the fight or flight response. Everyone, he concluded, can experience the relaxation response with training and motivation.

There are other paths to meditation. Western religion has its meditation; the rosary of the Roman Catholic Church is a long meditative prayer that has brought solace and comfort to millions of people for centuries. It is in widespread use today in many parts of the world.

Modern meditations also include mindfulness. In mindfulness, one focuses on living the day in full awareness rather than "going through the motions" of our daily lives as many of us do. Mindfulness can be part of the Yoga of Action, which teaches moderation, kindness and positiveness.

How to begin:
Seek out a quiet place where you will not be disturbed.
Sit in erect position, relaxed.
Breathe through the nose. Mouth is closed.
Close your eyes and with your mind's eye, follow your breath.
Do not change the breath.
Inhale, pause a moment, then exhale.
On the exhale, say the word "One" silently to yourself.
Pause a moment, repeat until you reach the count of five, then start over, with the count of one. When other thoughts intrude, let them pass by, as

a leaf might float down a mountain stream, not resisting the thought; then gently bring the mind back to the breath.

You need not use the word "One". You can reflect, contemplate on any subject that will help you relax.

At first try meditating for three minutes twice a day, eventually extending the time to 10 or 20 minutes twice a day.

As always, listen to your body. Do not ever force your body or mind in yoga or meditation.

When you are done, remain seated a few minutes, to savor the quiet, while the body changes from a quiet state to the ready state. Then stand up and resume the day's journey.

An Alternative, Simple, Equally Effective Meditation

Sit quietly, back straight in a chair or on your bed.
Close the eyes.
Count from 1 to 112.

This meditation is ancient although still in use. If prayer beads would help you meditate, go to a bead shop and ask for a string of wooden beads with 111 medium size beads and one large bead at the end, to signify stop. When finished, remain in a quiet state a few moments then stretch, stand up and continue your day. I find this meditation particularly effective in mid-evening or before Bedtime.

CHAPTER 12

Visualization, An Aid

To cut stress and give your life coherence from day to day, it is a good idea to visualize a map of your day.

Take a few moments after the morning stretches to sit quietly and picture in your mind's eye working with confidence to complete each task that is part of the day before you. Do this visualization with awareness and conviction. Then, at day's end, take another quiet moment to review. Tell yourself you did your best to meet your responsibilities that day.

This sort of informal, private time, a visualized day plan and later positive feedback or self pat on the back, if you will, I have found very helpful. Visualization gets me through the day easier; I am more truly my real self with other people and also to myself. When for some reason I don't do the visualization, I miss it. It makes the day more friendly and satisfying at both ends of the time span, as if your day at its core, belongs to you.

Most Americans are too hard on themselves. Women, especially, who meet demands of other people at home for long hours in addition to working jobs outside the home, have harder lives than ever these days. Researchers in behavioral psychology have found that women historically in primitive times have had a work life as well as a nurturing family life, but that present day job sites are unfriendly to the family in many, many ways. Such a work place causes excruciating stress in women with children. And yet, despite such heroic efforts women often feel they have done neither their work-job nor their home-job well. Not so! Give yourself credit for all that you are accomplishing!

Yoga Postures

Katie, Cabrillo College Student, Weight Trainer

1. Beginning Pose (Sit Pose).

2. Beginning Pose.

2b. Arm, shoulder, neck muscle stretch.

3. Thigh and leg muscles stretch, as you raise, lower thighs.

4. Neck, back stretch (firms jaw, face, neck muscles).

5. Beginning of reverse posture.

6. Reverse posture (circultaion aid for entire body; brain gets fresh blood, thinking clears).

7. |Back stretch–neck reversed from posture 4, firming, stretching different face muscles; brings fresh blood to face, improves skin tone.

8. Do not do this pose or attempt it unless you have done yoga for at least 6 months to a year. Back must be in shape.

9. See instruction 7.

10. Reverse of posture 6 with all reverse benefits.

11. Warrior pose–strengthens entire body; excellent for balance*

12. Cross-legged pose, holding toes; prepare for back roll.

13. After back roll.

14. Ending pose (child pose). Calming, nurturing. Let go…

* This is one of my additions to Charles Horn's invaluable everyday work-
out series. It is of course the warrior pose. Almost immediately strength-
ening, invaluable for those with poor posture, it directly affects leg, arm
and hip strength. Hold to count of 10, or beginners, judge when fatigue
sets in; then stop.

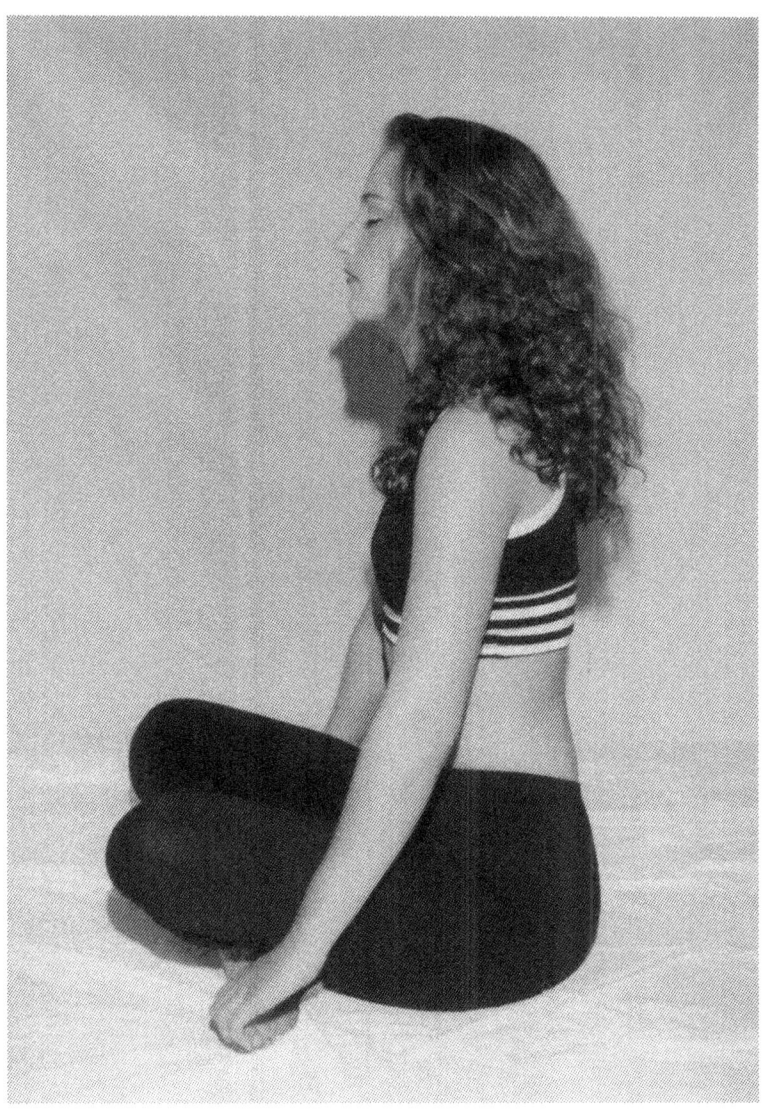

1. Beginning Pose (Sit-Pose)

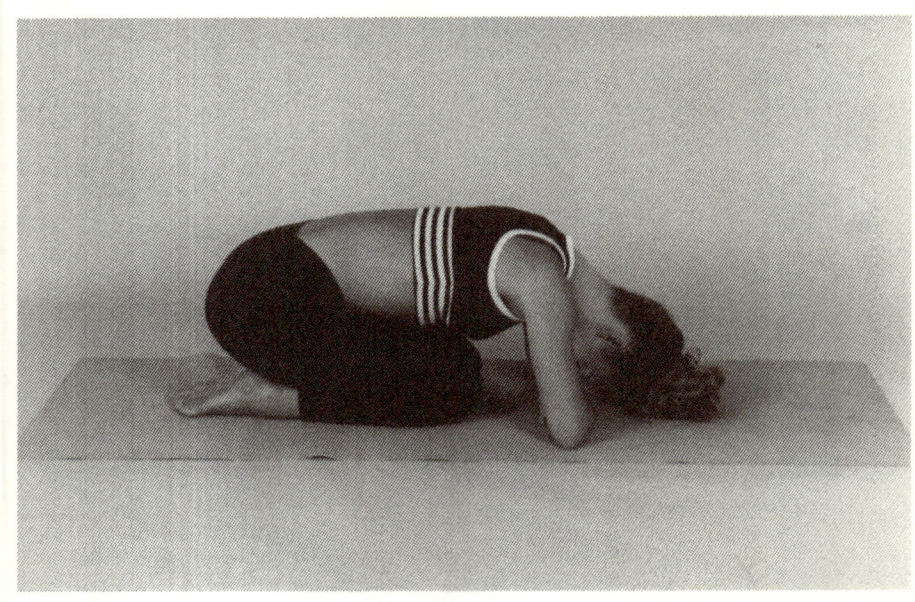

2. Beginning pose.

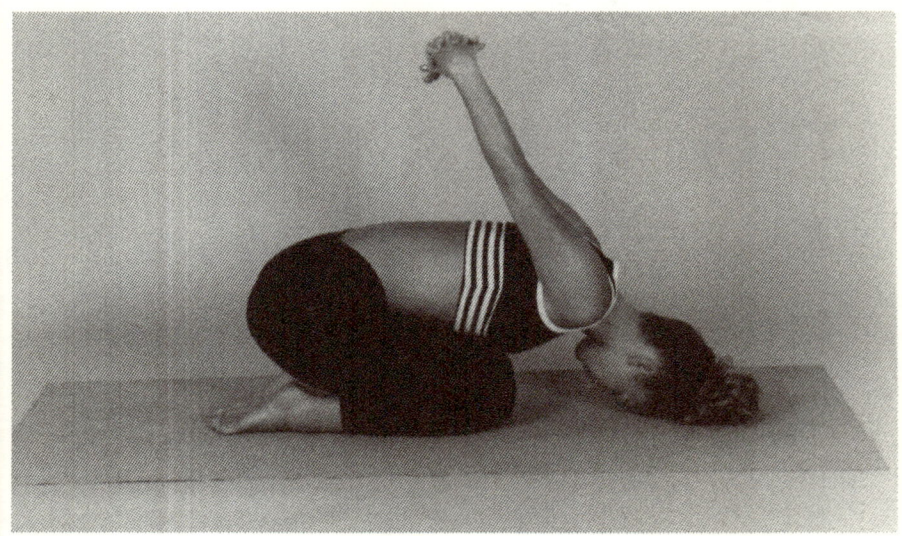

2b. Arm, shoulder, neck muscle stretch..

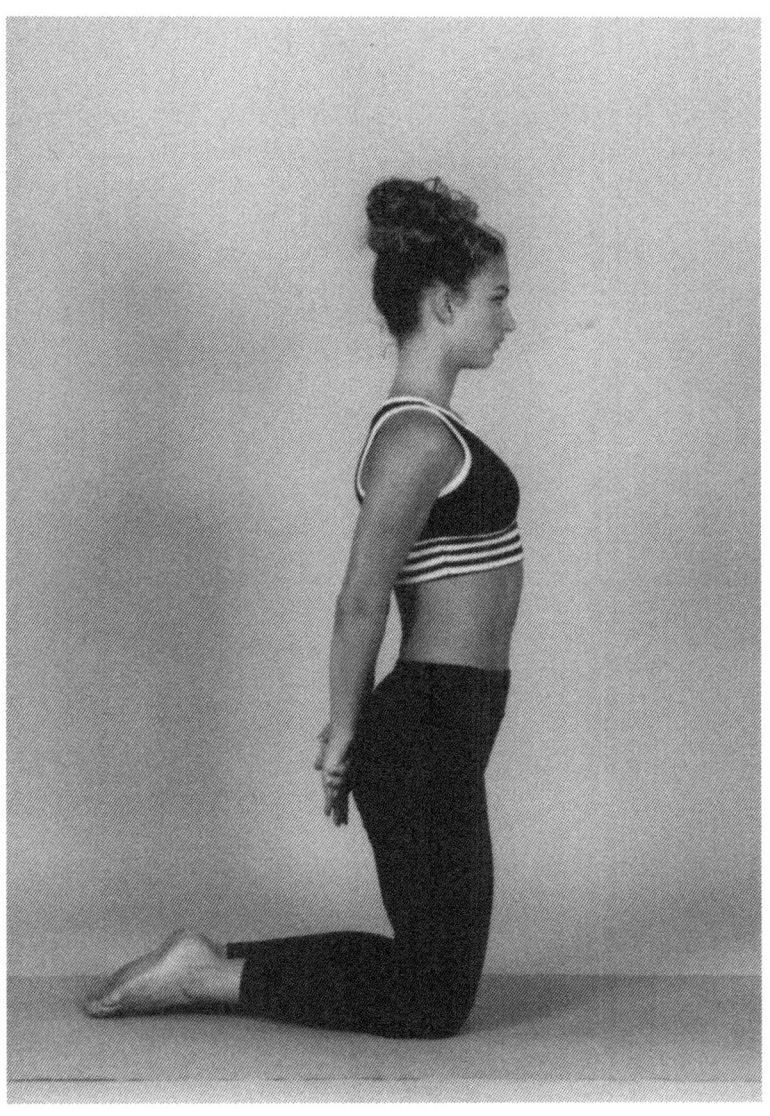

3. Thigh and leg muscles stretch, as you raise, lower thighs.

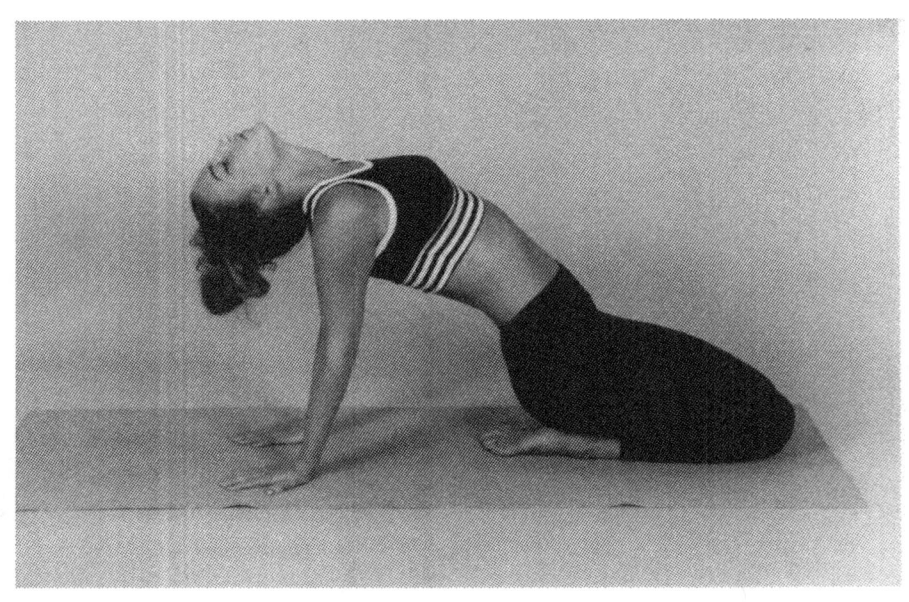

4. Neck, back stretch (firms jaw, face, neck muscles).

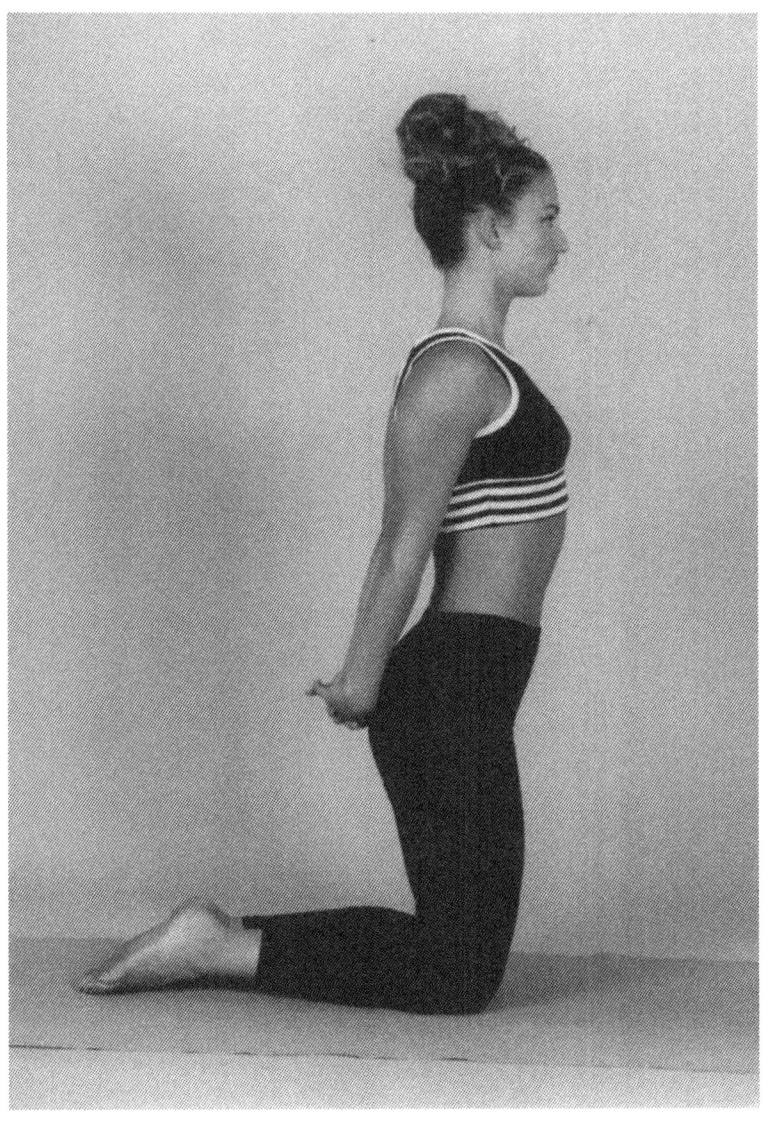

5. Beginning of reverse posture.

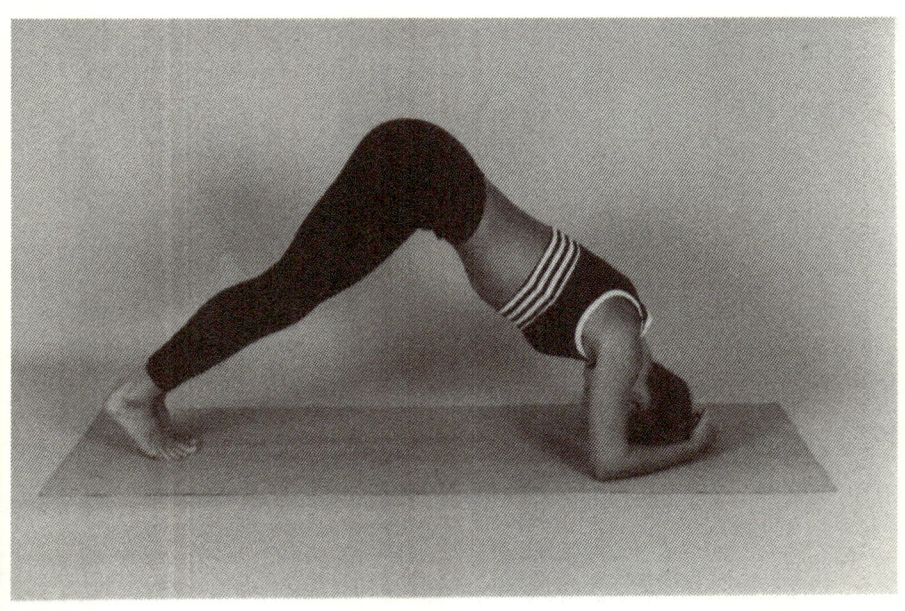

6. Reverse posture (circultaion aid for entire body; brain gets fresh blood, thinking clears).

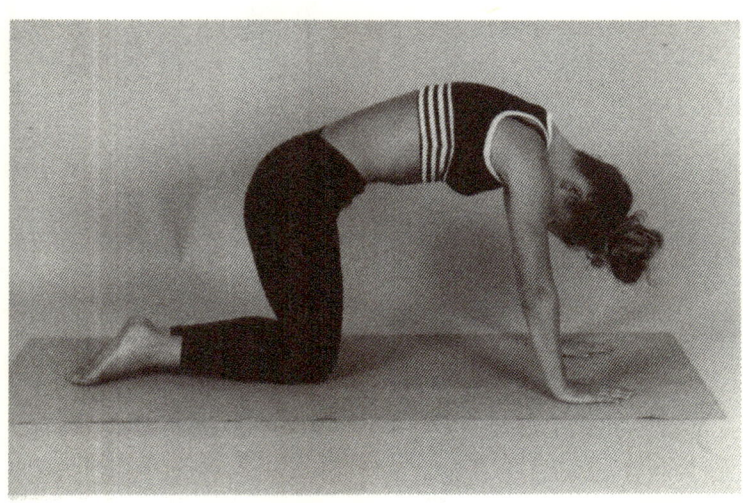

7. Back stretch—neck reversed from posture 4, firming, stretching different face muscles; brings fresh blood to face, improves skin tone.

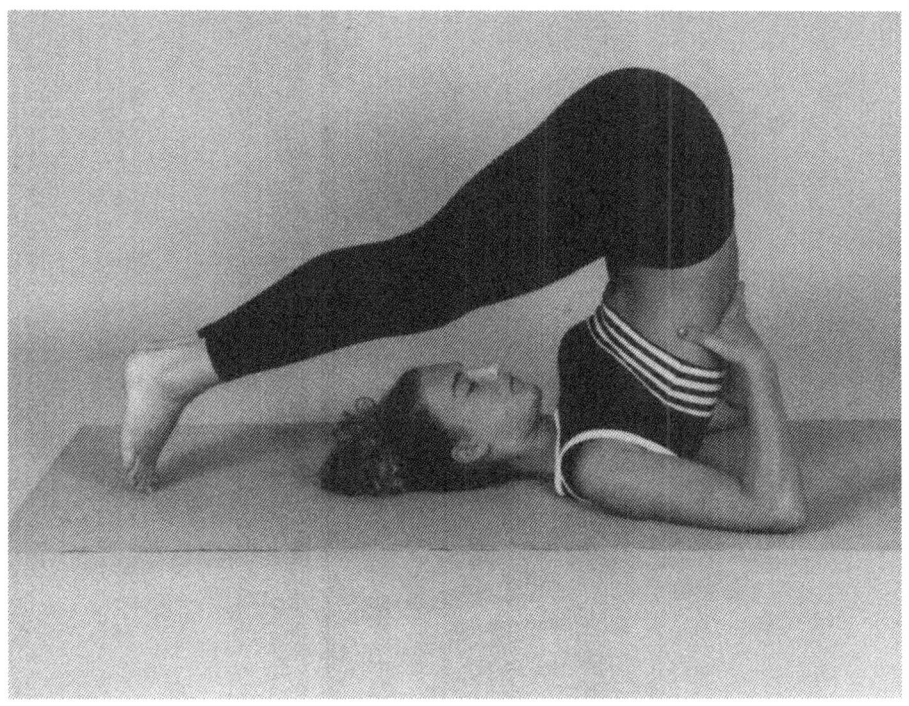

*8. Do not do this pose or attempt it unless you have done yoga for at least 6 months to a year. Back **must** be in shape.*

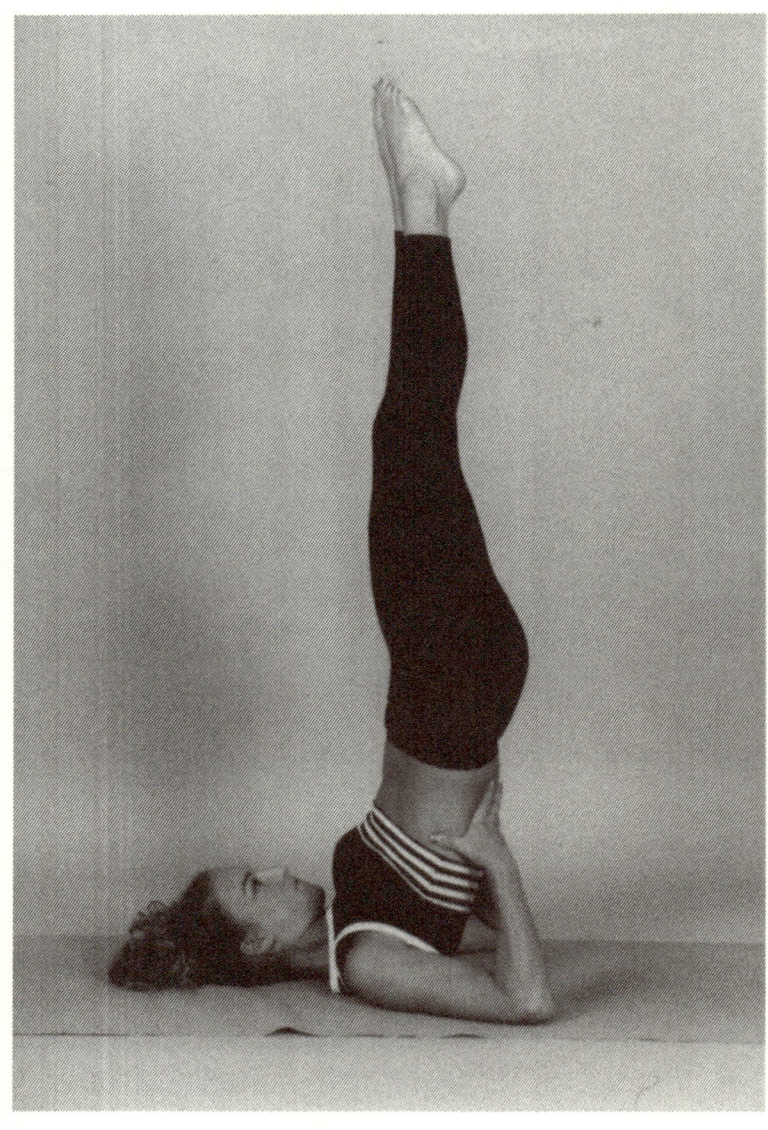

9. See instruction 7.

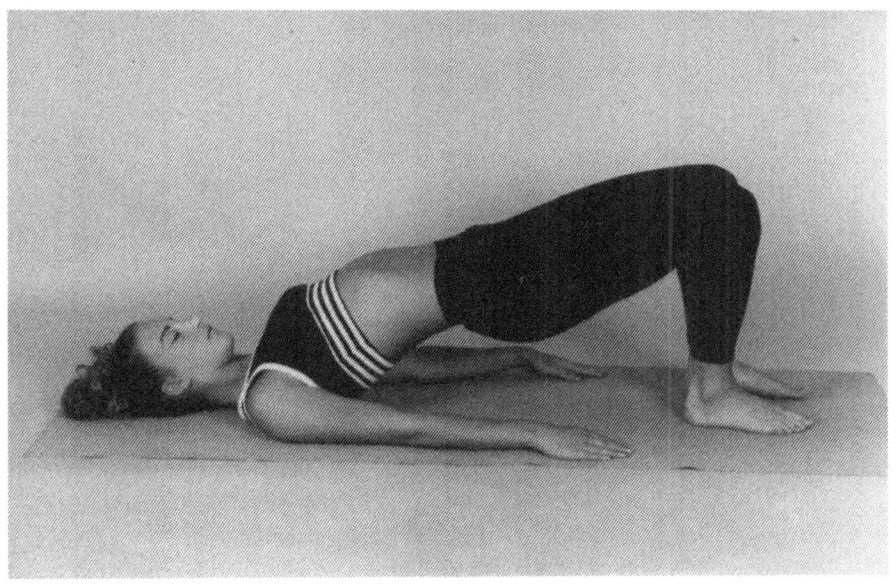

10. Reverse of posture 6 with all the reverse benefits.

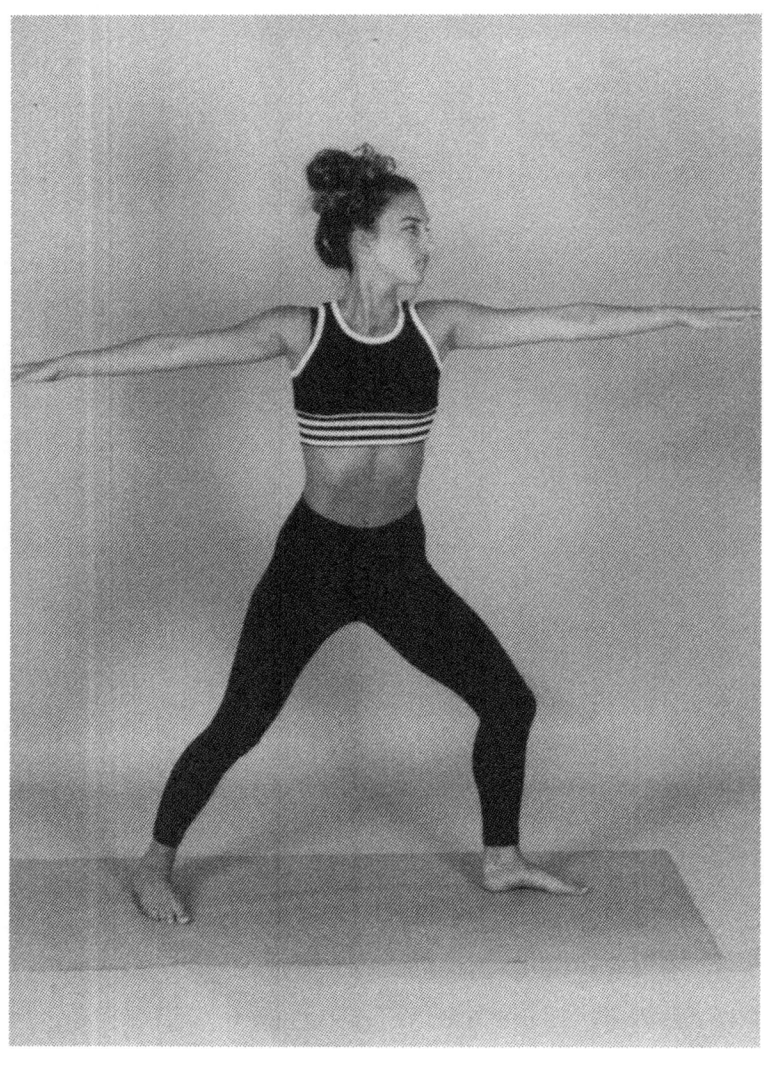

11. Warrior pose–strengthens entire body; excellent for balance*

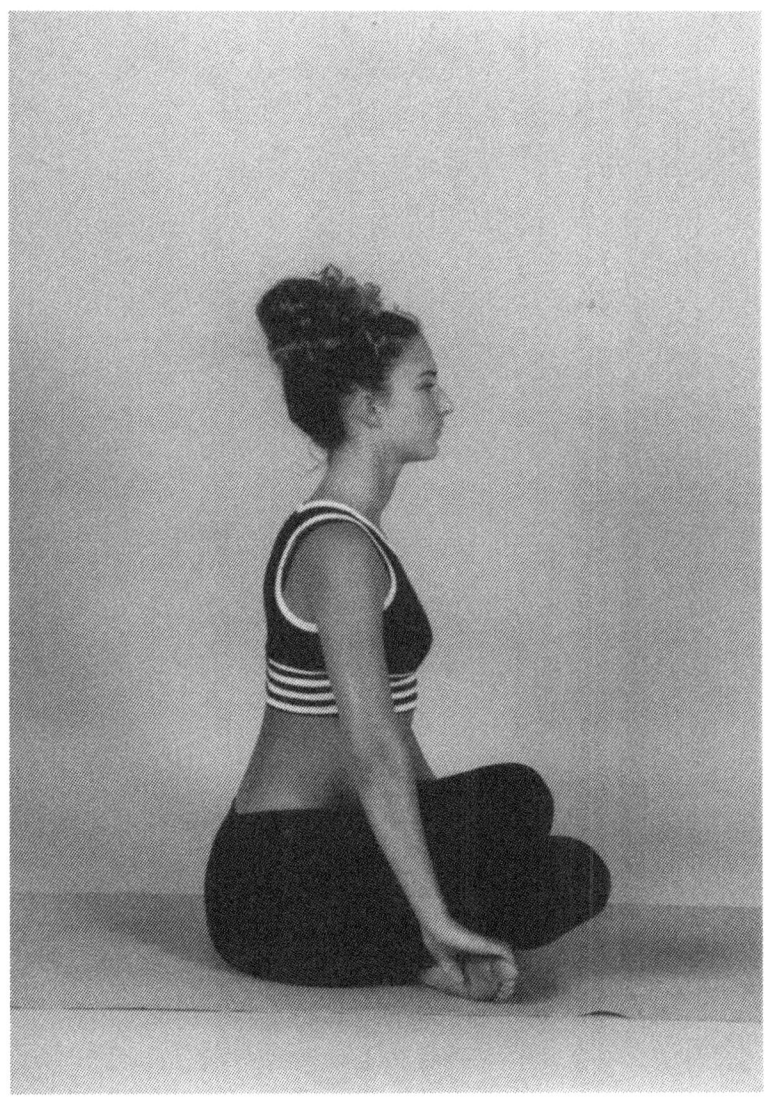

12. Cross-legged pose, holding toes; prepare for back roll.

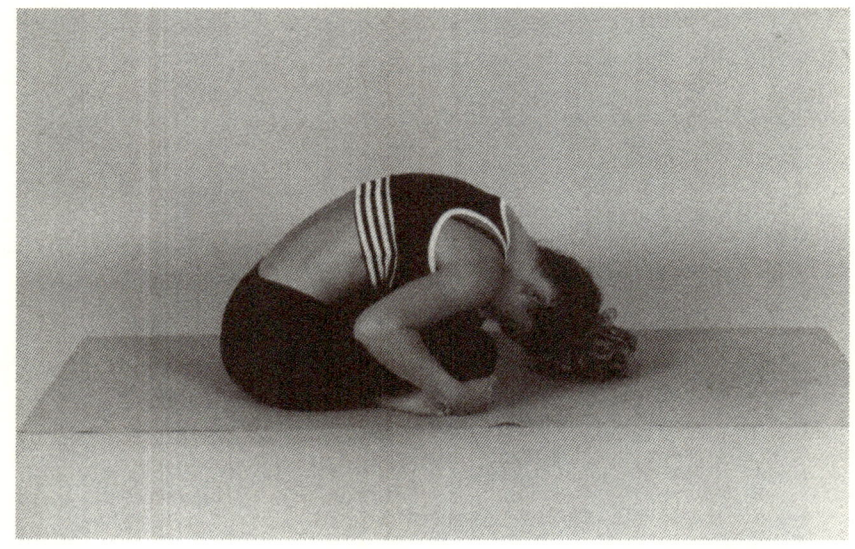

13. After back roll.

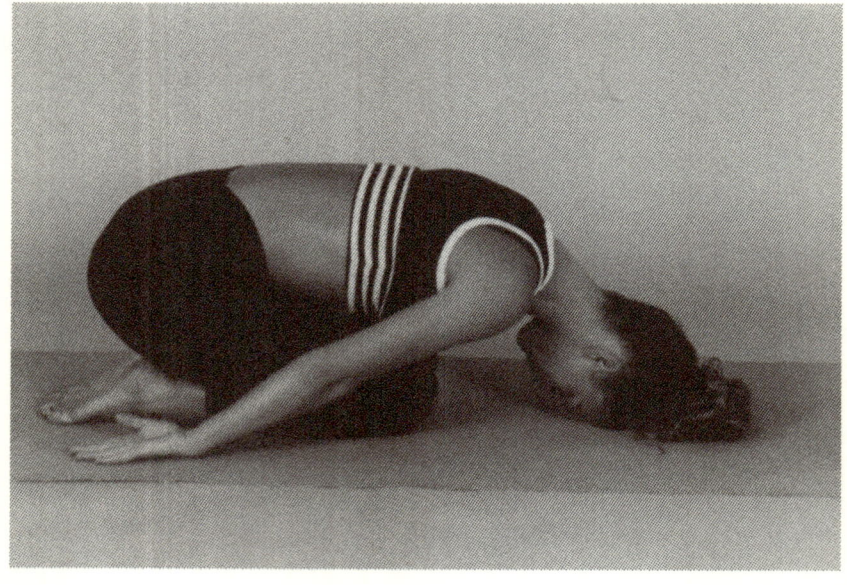

14. Ending pose (child pose). Calming, nurturing. Let go...

Yoga Postures

Yvonne, Author

1. Muscles in the arm, hip, thigh, knee, neck are stretched.

2. Back, shoulders, arm stretches.

3. Balance pose (mild) arm, shoulder, muscle stretch.

4. Neck, chin muscle stretch; leg, back, neck muscle stretch.

5. Anyone over 30 needs this! Achilles stretch and leg stretch. Leg should be straight (after practice). See pose 9.

5a. Count leg extension. Note leg is straight.

6. Preparation for balance leg stretch, chin to knee neck muscle stretch.

7. Right leg balance stretch. (Medium-difficult balance pose.)

8. Preparation for Left leg balance stretch. (Note position of heads, hands, toes, ankle.)(Foot muscle stretch.)

9. Achilles tendon and leg muscle, ankle tendon stretch. Note foot position. Dip foot very gently toward you, then away from you. Good for runners.

10. Warrior pose. Feel stronger fast!

11. Beginning calming pose.

12. Continued calming pose. Roll to the right.

13. Calming pose: roll to left then back to center.

13a. Roll back to center. Then assume child pose. See next page.

14. Child pose, (See Katie series, number 14.)

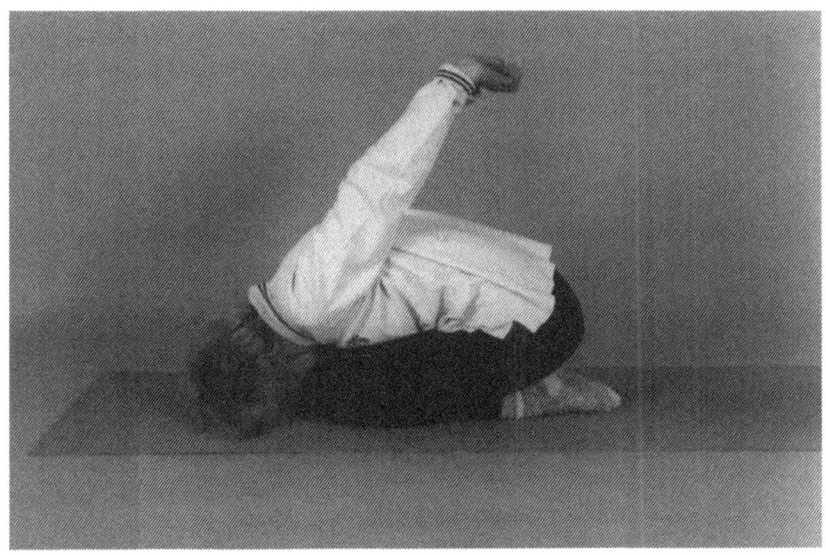

1. Muscles in the arm, hip, thigh, knee, neck are stretched.

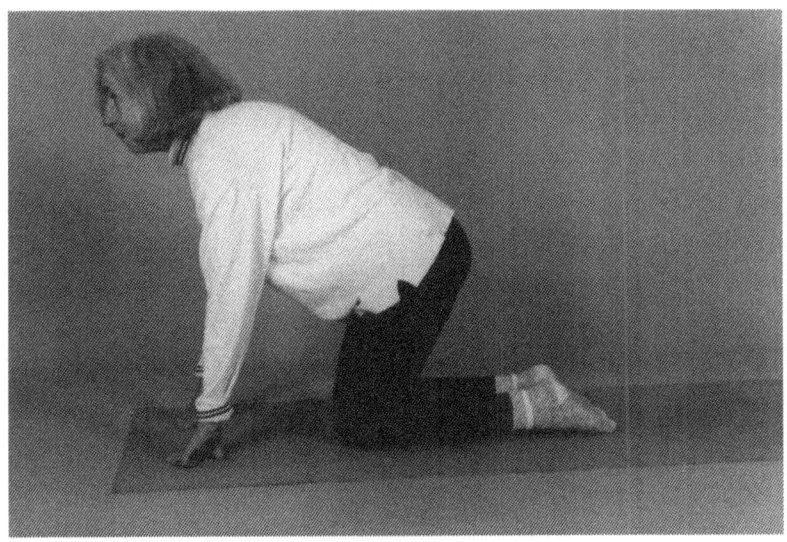

2. Back, shoulders, arm stretches.

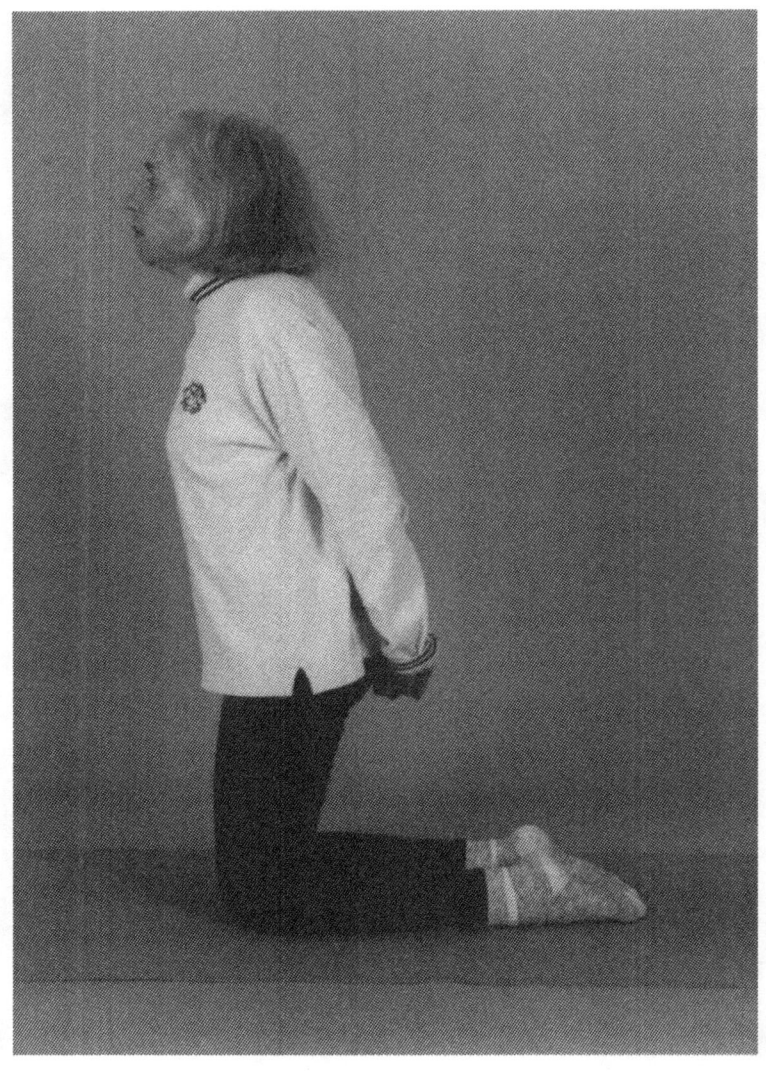

3. Balance pose (mild) arm, shoulder, muscle stretch.

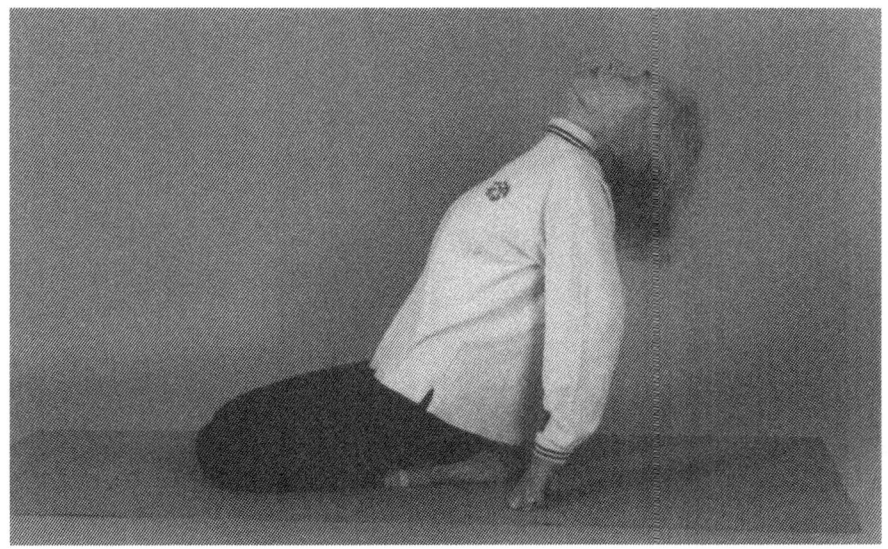

4. *Neck, chin muscle stretch; leg, back, neck muscle stretch.*

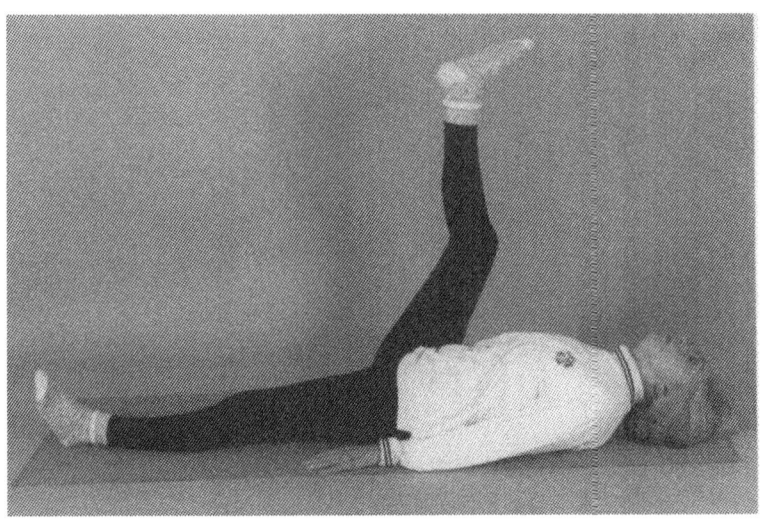

5. *Anyone over 30 needs this! Achilles stretch and leg stretch. Leg should be straight (after practice). See pose 5a*

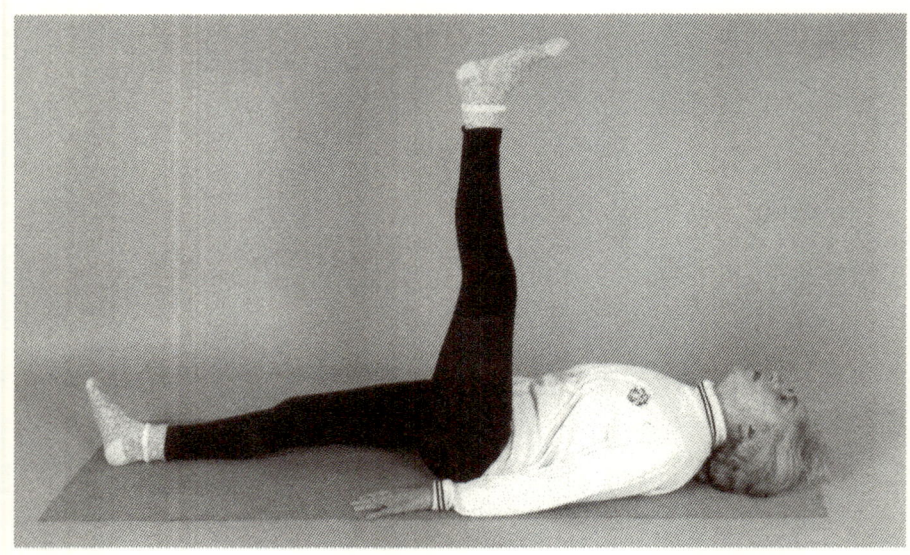

5a. Corect leg extension. Note leg is straight.

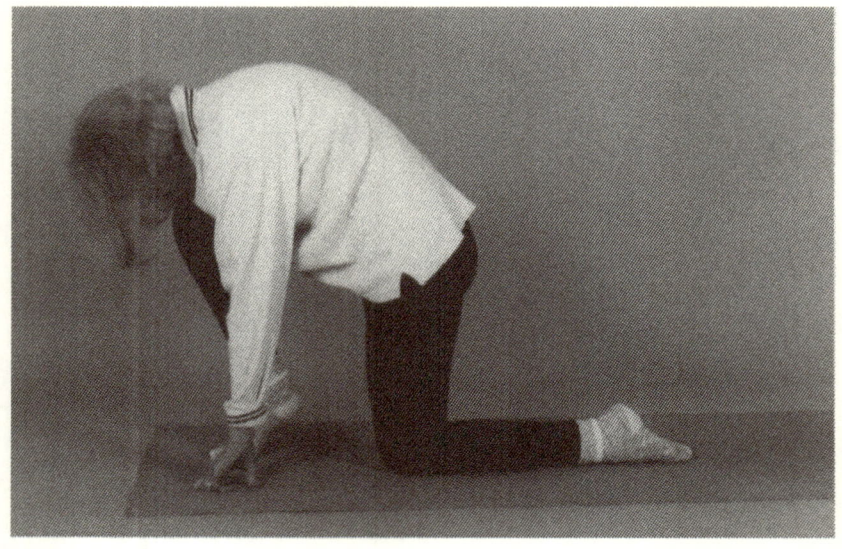

6. Preparation for balance leg stretch, chin to knee neck muscle stretch.

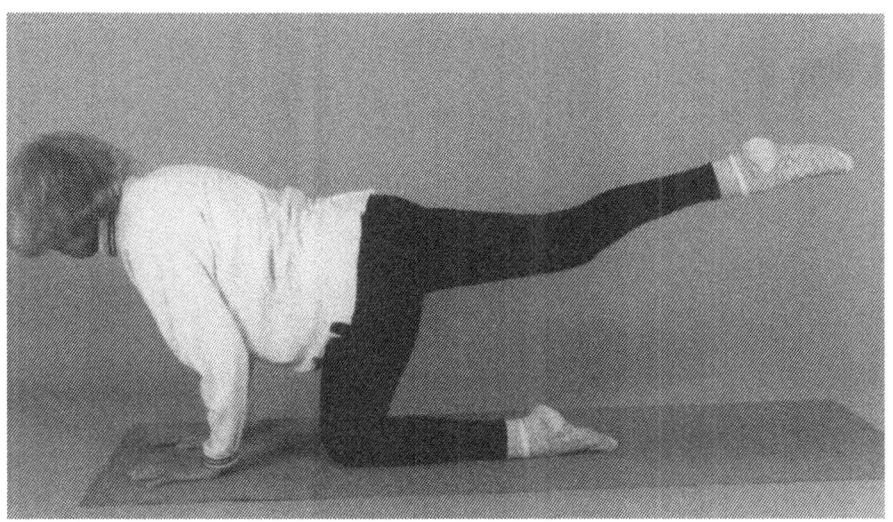

7. Right leg balance stretch. (Medium-difficult balance pose.)

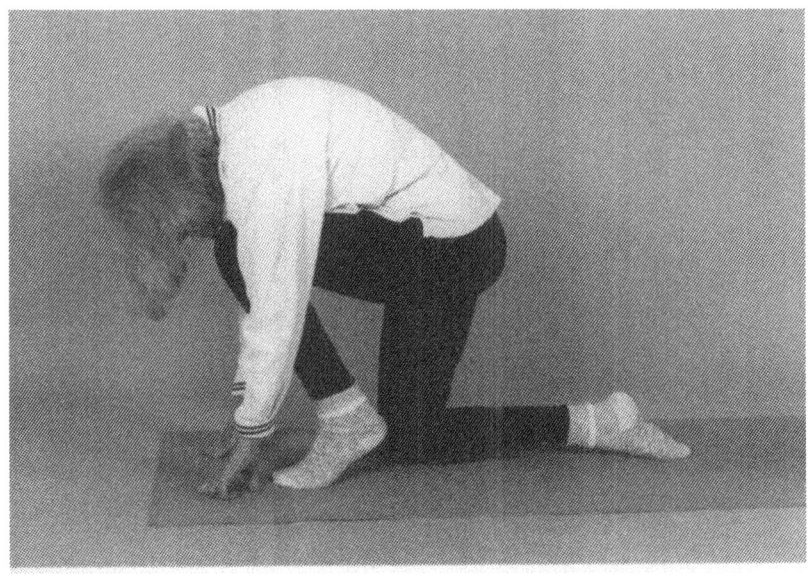

8. Preparation for Left leg balance stretch. (Note position of head, hands, toes, ankle.)(Foot muscle stretch.)

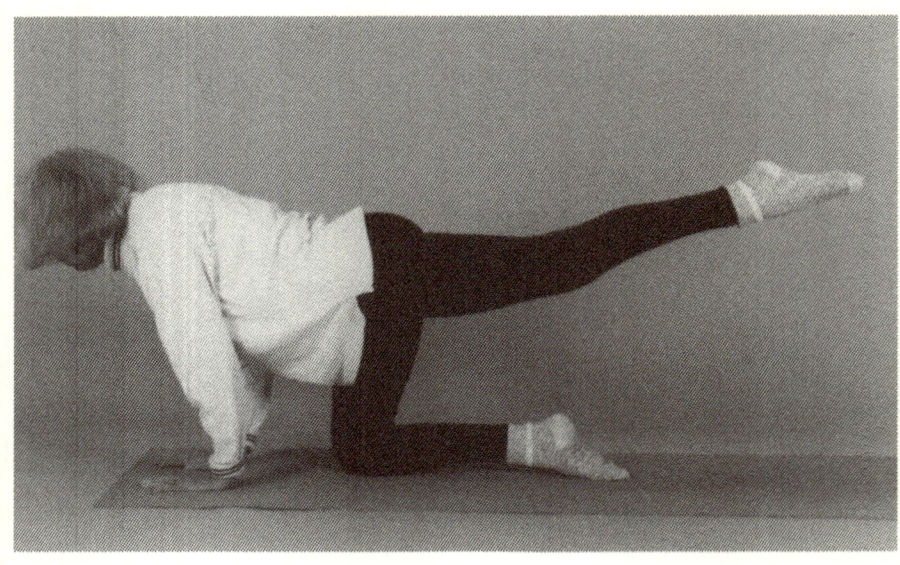

9. Achilles tendon and leg muscle, ankle tendon stretch. Note foot position. Dip foot very gently toward you, then away from you. Good for runners.

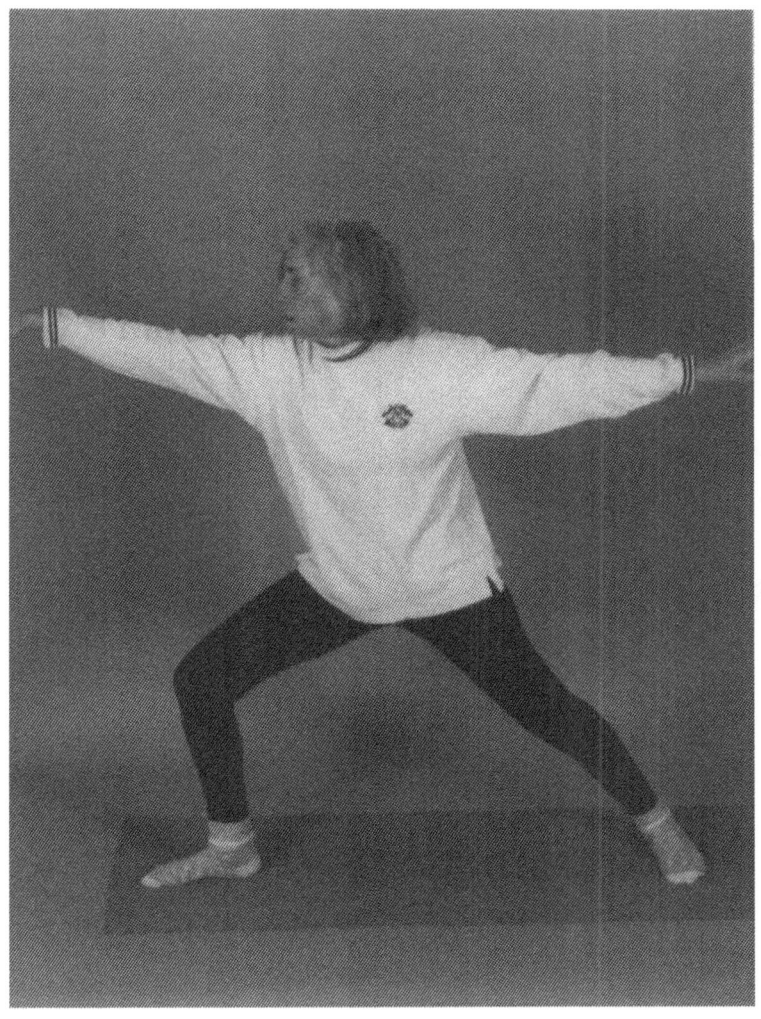

10. Warrior pose. Feel stronger fast!

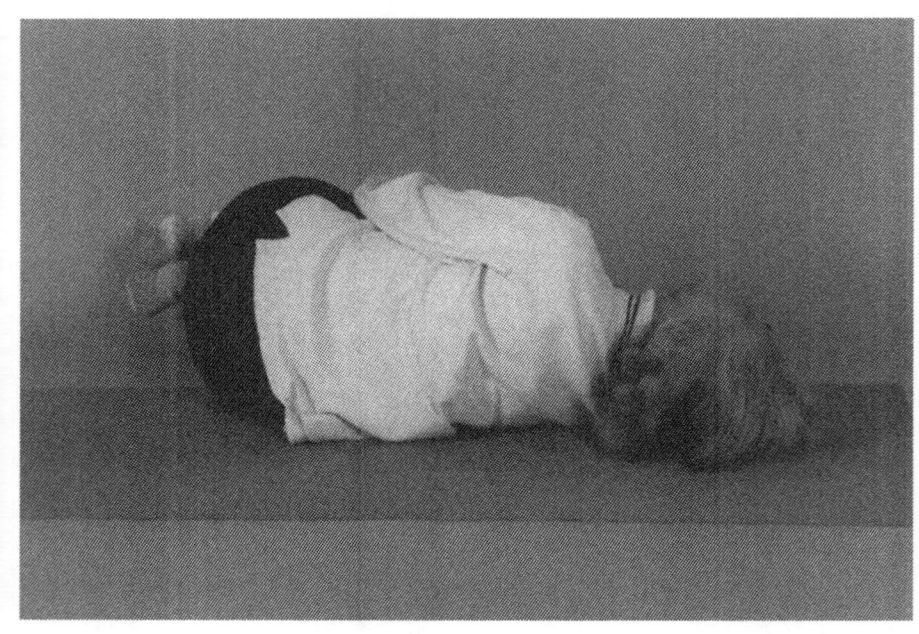

11. Calming pose: roll to left then back to center.

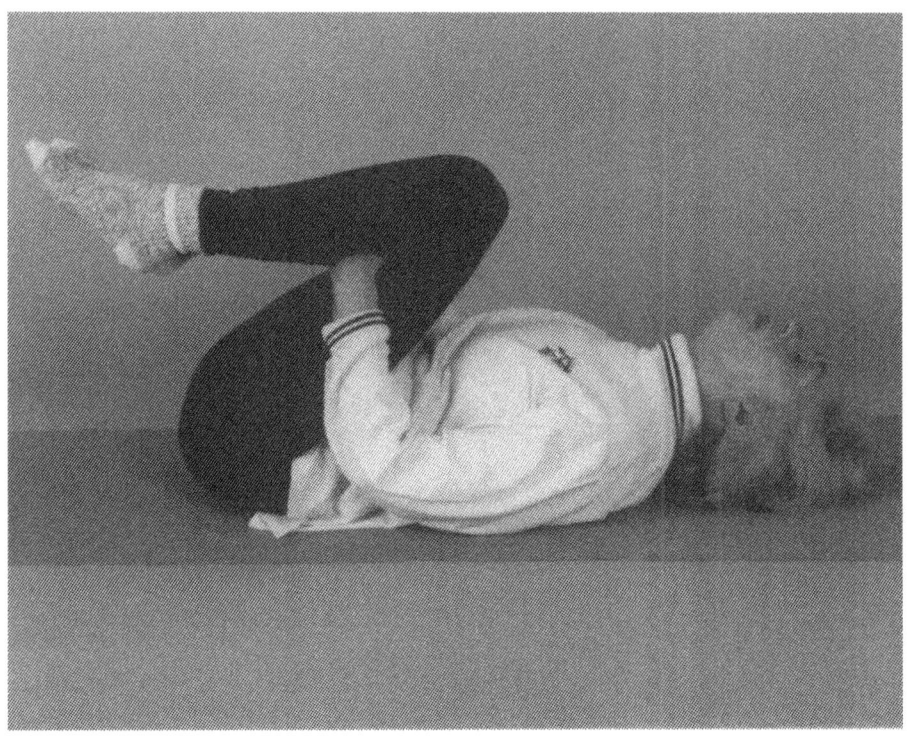

12. Continued calming pose. Back to center then, Roll to the right.

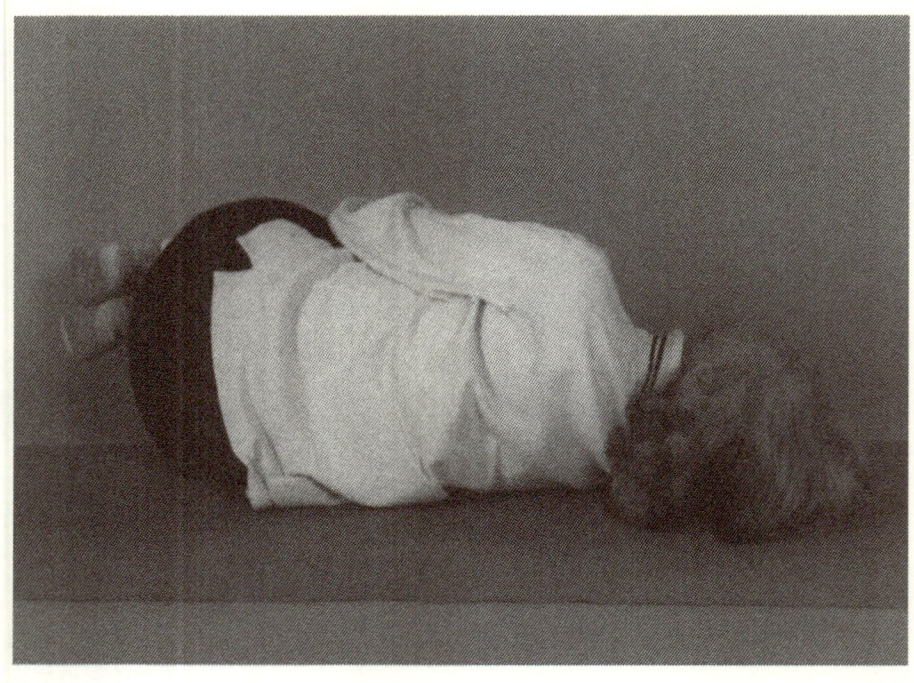

13. Calming pose: roll to left then back to center.

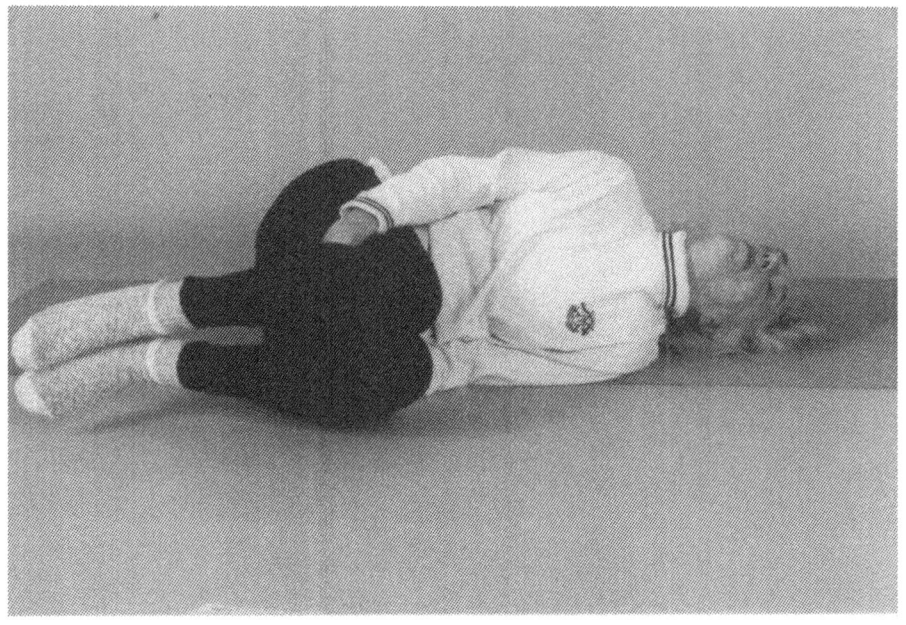

13a. Roll back to center. Then assume child pose. See next page.

14. Child pose, (See Katie series, number 14.)

BIBLIOGRAPHY

The Second Fifty Years: Promoting Health and Preventing Disability, U.S. Institute of Medicine. National Academy Press, National Academy of Sciences, Washington, D.C.

We Live Too Short and Die Too Long, Walter M. Bortz, M.D. Bantam Books, 1991. (Paperback also)

How and Why We Age, Leonard Hayflick, Ph.D., Ballantine Books, a Division of Random House, 1994.

Health After Fifty, Johns Hopkins Health Letter. Monthly newsletter from the University Medical School, housing the nation's #1 rated hospital.

Healthwise Handbook. subtitled *"A Self-Care Manual For You And Your Family,* Twelfth edition, 1995, Healthwise Publications, P.O. Box 1989, Boise, ID 83701 (208) 345-1161. (Group Health Cooperative of Puget Sound at Virginia Mason Hospital, Seattle, WA.) This is a sensible, comprehensive, humane book for lay people. Easy reading, easy to grasp text and index. Highly recommended.

Be Young and Flexible After 30, 40, 50, 60...., Ruth Bender, Ruben Publishing, Avon, CT, 1976. P.O. Box 414, Avon, CT 06001. An excellent book to pick up as a refresher any time that you cannot walk or do yoga regularly.

Yoga for Common Ailments, Drs. Robin, Monroe, Nagarathna, Nagendra, Simon and Shuster, 1990, London. (Paper) A most beautiful yoga book, large color pictures, sketches, very useful text.

Office Yoga-Tackling Tension with Simple Stretches You Can Do at Your Desk, Julie Friedeberger, Thorsons, an Imprint of Harper Collins Publishers, 1992.

The Complete Illustrated Book of Yoga, Swami Vishnu Devandanda, Bell Publishing, a Division of Crown Publishers, by arrangement with the Julian Press, Inc. A classic.

Resiliency: How To Bounce Back Faster, Stronger, Smarter, Tessa Albert Warshaw, Ph.D. and Dee Barlow, Ph.D., Master Media, Limited.

Yoga for Americans, Indra Devi, Prentice Hall, 1959, Englewood Cliffs, NJ. An early book by the inspiring yoga icon, still beautiful, radiant, and now living in Mexico; a visitor to Santa Cruz not too long ago.

Harvard Women's Health Watch Newsletter, published monthly; Harvard Medical School Publications Group, 164 Longwood Avenue, Boston, MA 02115. Excellent index to articles issued yearly. Sponsors comprehensive reports issued various times during the year on current research in health matters affecting women of all ages. Reads easily. Clear.

Mind and Body Health Newsletter, The Center for Health Sciences c/o ISHK Book Service, P.O. Box 381069, Cambridge, MA 02234-1069, or call 1-800-222-4745. Concise, research-based. Fascinating and informative.

Easy Does It Yoga for Older People, Alice Christensen and David Rankin, The Light of Yoga Society, 1979, Harper & Row, New York, 1998 new edition available. Lots of good info. Style/content a mish-mash.

Family Guide to Natural Medicine, Reader's Digest, Pleasantville, NY, 1993. The Reader's Digest went well into the alternative medicine field and the result is interesting reading, excellent illustrations and quite comprehensive; a colorful read. Altogether satisfying.

The Healer Within: The Four Essential Self-Care Techniques for Creating Optimal Health, Roger Jahnke, Harper, San Francisco, 1997.

University of Texas Lifetime Health Letter, monthly newsletter published by the University of Texas-Houston Health Science Center, 7000 Famire DCT 212, Houston, Texas 77030. Excellent, informal (almost down-home at times) health letter covers broader than most in its field. Easy to read, accessible info for lay people. Its person-to-person style, lacking the usual academic paternalism, refreshing indeed.

Dr. Dean Ornish's Program for Reversing Heart Disease, by Dean Ornish, M.D., Ballantine Books, a division of Random House, Inc., New York, 1990. A pioneering book on a method that treats the whole person, by a courageous physician.

Spencer, G, Projections of the population by age, race and sex-1983-2080. Current Population Reports, U.S. Bureau of the Census, Series P-25, No. 952, 1984.

Christian Yoga, Fr. Jean Déchanet, S.J., 1950(?). A seminal book on the subject for the author.

The Art and Practice of Loving, Frank Andrews, Ph.D., Jeremy Tarcher/Perigee, G.P. Putnam, 1991, 1992 (Paper)

Necessary Losses, Judith Viorst, 1986, Fawcett Gold Medal Books.

A World Waiting to Be Born, M. Scott Peck, M.D., A Bantam Book, 1993. A wonderful book on community and how to build it. Easy to read, compassionate, innovative look at our world in the U.S. Healing words and ideas.

True Yoga, William Zorn, A. Thomas and Co., London, 1966; Wehman and Co., Pub. Hackensack, NJ. Inspiring story of yoga by a prisoner of war who survived captivity because of yoga's benefits.

Be Young with Yoga, Richard L.Hittleman,Paper Library, Coronet Communications, New York, 1971. Classic Hittleman.

The Journal of Alternative and Complementary Medicine, Mary Ann Liebert, Inc., Publishers, 1651-Fifth Ave., New York 10128.

Healing Mind, Healthy Woman, Alice Domar and Henry Dreher, Henry Holt, 1997. Domar is director of women's health programs at Harvard Medical School, Division of Behavioral Medicine. Practical mind-body strategies for relieving stress/building health.

The Anatomy of the Spirit, Carolyn Myss, Ph.D. An attempt to link Eastern and Western views of the Spirit, not always successful, always quirky and interesting.

Yoga Journal, 2054 University Avenue, Berkeley, CA 94074. Excellent respected source for Yoga books, teachers and ideas for the yoga life.

The Asian Journal of Thomas Merton, New Directions Paperback, 1975, New Directions Publishing Corporation, New York. A rich experience in reading and thinking.

A Book of Psalms, selected and adapted from the Hebrew, 85pp, Stephen Mitchell, Harper Perennial, a Division of Harper Collins Publishers. The author rewrites the Psalms (!) and succeeds at it.

Touching the Holy, Ordinariness, Self-Esteem and Friendship, Robert J. Wicks, Ave Maria Press, Notre Dame, Indiana, 1992. A book intended for pastors by a counselor to those professionals, works equally well for the inquiring reader. Astringent thinking, good writing. A different tack on how the human spirit grows and thrives, written with a caring pen.

SELECTED RESOURCES INCLUDING WEBSITES*

* indicates website

Aging. National Institute on Aging. 1-800-222-2225 (8:30-5 ET)

Alcohol and Drug Abuse. National clearinghouse for alcohol and drug info. 1-800-729-6686 (8-7 ET) Includes information on tobacco, all clearinghouse material comes from either the Center for Substance Abuse Prevention, National Institute on Drug Abuse or National Institute on Alcohol Abuse and Alcoholism.

Allergy. National Institute of Allergy and Infectious Diseases. 301-496-5717 (8:30-5 ET)

*Alternative Medicine. Global Navigator's Alternative Medicine Sites. http:/www.gna/com/wic/wics/alt/html

Alzheimer's Disease. Alzheimer's Association. 1-800-272-3900 (8-5 Central time)

American Dietetic Association *Nutrition Hotline* 1-800-366-1655. Referrals, experts. (8-8 Central time)

*America Online. This much-favored health discussion group now on the web.

Some topics open for chat not covered by experts or M.D.s
(*www.betterhealth.com*)

American Heart Association. 1-800-242-8721

American Psychiatric Association 202-682-6000

American Psychological Association 202-336-5500

American Association for Marriage & Family Therapy 1-800-822-3000

American Psychiatric Nurses Association 202-857-1133

Arthritis. Arthritis Foundation 1-800-283-7800 (24-hour recording)

Cancer. Information Service of the National Cancer Institute. 1-800-4-CANCER Cancerfax 1-800-674-2511 (24 hours) Source for current patient and professional information on all types of cancer, sponsored by above institute.

*Centers for Disease Control and Prevention (http://www.cdc.gov/) 404-332-4555, 24-hour recording and phone 8-4:30 ET.

Chronic Fatigue Syndrome. CFIDS Association. 1-800-442-3437 (24-hour recording)

Deafness and Communication Disorders. National Institute on *Deafness* and Other Communication Disorders. 1-800-241-1044 (8:15-5 ET) 1-800-241-1055 (TDD/TTY/TT) Hearing impaired telephones available so deaf can call.

Dentistry. National Institute of Dental Research. 301-496-4261. (8:30 A.M.–5:00 P.M. ET)

Depression Awareness. 1-800-421-4211 (24-hour recording) Hotline discusses symptoms and treatment of depression.

Drug Evaluation and Research. 301-827-4573 (9-4:30 ET) Hotline sponsored by U.S. Food and Drug Administration gives info about medicines.

Fibromyalgia Alliance of America 614-457-4222 (24-hour recording plus daily attended phone line)

Grief Recovery Helpline. Reference Grief Recovery Handbook, James and Friedman. Harper Collins. Grief counseling is accessible via local Hospice sites. Sudden death counseling is extremely helpful. Local Humane Societies sometimes offer counseling for the death of pets.

Incontinence. The Simon Foundation for Continence Newsletter and other publications. 1-800-237-4466.

*Internet. Mental Health Home Page (**http://www.mentalhealth-comm/p.html**)

*Johns Hopkins University/Aetna Healthcare Joint approach. Includes "Ask-the-Doc" time with University physicians. (**www.betterhealth.com**)

*Dr. C. Everett Koop, N.S.,M.D. Former surgeon general's site (**www.koop.com**)
Includes interactive portion with panels of medical experts supervising.

Lung Problems. American Lung Association.
1-800-LUNG-USA (9-4:30 ET) Lung disease information. Don't smoke.

*The Melpomine Institute for Women's Health Research. Non-profit, Minneapolis-based institute researches health-related issues affecting physically active women, i.e. osteoporosis and menopause. Named for the first woman marathon runner. The Melpomine Institute, 1010 University Ave. West, St. Paul, MN 55104. 651-642-1951. Website (http:/www.melpomine.org)
has info re: health questions of physically active girls/women, exercise during pregnancy, etc.National Association of Social Workers 1-800-638-8799

*Menopause–Midlife Women's Network 1-800-886-4354 (8-5 Central time) Info and referrals.

*Menopause. North American Menopause Society
(http:/www.menopause.com)

*National Eye Institute. 301-496-5248 (8:00 A.M. –5:00 P.M. ET)

*The New England Journal of Medicine (http://www.nejm.org) Excellent medical research journal. Most articles very technical; online site more easily accessible, offering abstracts of current journal articles, research opportunities by topic or author in past issues. Journal has unveiled much ground-breaking research in its pages over the past 15 years.

Psychotherapy/Mental Health Information. National Alliance for the Mentally Ill
1-800-950-6264. Good source for general information on mental illness.

Sex Questions. Albert Ellis Institute, 45 E. 65th St., New York, 10021. Provides information on sex and problems with sex at a reasonable fee. Ellis was a pioneer sex researcher of 50 years ago or so who was well-respected by the scientific community, unlike Masters and Johnson.

Stroke. American Heart Association Stroke Connection 1-800-553-6321 (8:30-5 Central time) Newsletter. Information by phone, referrals.

*University of California, San Francisco. ***www.shn.net*** University of California Medical School (San Francisco) website features M.D.s/nurses as online experts during chats. ***www.shn.net***.

University of Washington, Northwest Prevention Effectiveness Center, Seattle, WA. The only federally funded program doing on-going research in simple, effective ways of health promotion in people over 65. Low-tech methods, hand weights, water exercises in this program illustrate the simple effectiveness of moving, as stressed in *Yoga and Optimum Health after 40.* The striking social benefits of exercise programs also monitored here. University of Washington Medical School, Seattle, Washington.

www.ingramcontent.com/pod-product-compliance
Lightning Source LLC
Chambersburg PA
CBHW020253290526
45784CB00003B/1231